Optimizing Therapy Dog-Handler Team Welfare

Informed by research and grounded in critical discussions of theory and practice, *Optimizing Therapy Dog-Handler Team Welfare* challenges readers to explore the complexities inherent in, and arising from, practices that optimize welfare for therapy dog-handler teams.

Each chapter begins with a case study that elucidates the complexities of canine-assisted interventions and invites readers to consider welfare from multiple perspectives. This book positions welfare as a factor impacting both the therapy dog and the handler, considering the dog handler as a cohesive team.

Researchers, educators, and practitioners from across disciplines will find this book both scientifically savvy and practical.

John-Tyler Binfet, PhD, is a professor in the Faculty of Education at the University of British Columbia, Okanagan campus.

Christine Yvette Tardif-Williams, PhD, is a professor in the Department of Child and Youth Studies at Brock University.

JOHN-TYLER BINFET
AND CHRISTINE YVETTE
TARDIF-WILLIAMS

Optimizing Therapy Dog-Handler Team Welfare

A Guide for Researchers and Practitioners

Routledge
Taylor & Francis Group

NEW YORK AND LONDON

Designed cover image: Freya L. L. Green Photography; used with permission.

First published 2026
by Routledge
605 Third Avenue, New York, NY 10158

and by Routledge
4 Park Square, Milton Park, Abingdon, Oxon, OX14 4RN

Routledge is an imprint of the Taylor & Francis Group, an informa business

ISBN: 978-1-032-63797-6 (hbk)
ISBN: 978-1-032-63798-3 (pbk)
ISBN: 978-1-032-63928-4 (ebk)

DOI: 10.4324/9781032639284

Typeset in Joanna MT
by codeMantra

We dedicate this book to all the hard-working therapy dogs and handlers who bring joy to clients in programmes around the world. May the contents of our book help ensure their well-being.

Contents

List of Figures and Tables

TABLES

Declaration of generative artificial intelligence (AI) and AI-assisted technologies in the writing process. Neither AI nor AI-assisted technologies were used in the planning, design, or writing of this manuscript.

Appreciation

Our ability throughout this manuscript to provide readers with rich visual representations of concepts and interactions was made possible by the talents and insights of Ms. Freya Green. We are grateful for her keen eye and knowledge of canine-assisted interventions.

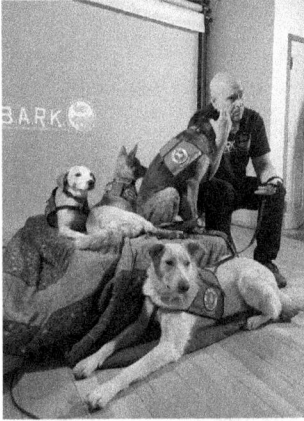

John-Tyler Binfet, PhD, is a professor in the Faculty of Education at the University of British Columbia (UBC), Okanagan campus. His research explores prosocial behaviour in children and adolescents and the effects of canine-assisted interventions on college student well-being. He is the author of three previous books including the recently co-authored *Virtual Human-Animal Interactions: Supporting Learning, Social Connections and Well-Being* (Tardif-Williams & Binfet, 2023; Routledge), *Cultivating Kindness: An Educator's Guide* (2022; University of Toronto Press), and the co-authored *Canine-Assisted Interventions: A Comprehensive Guide to Credentialing Therapy Dog Teams* (Binfet & Hartwig, 2020; Routledge). His research on the effects of canine-assisted interventions has been published in *Anthrozoös,* the *Journal of Mental Health, Human-Animal Interactions,* and the *Journal of Veterinary Behavior,* among elsewhere. He is the founder and director of UBC's *Building Academic Retention through K9s* (B.A.R.K.) program, established in 2012, which routinely oversees 60+ therapy dogs and their handlers participating in on-campus and community programming.

Dr. Binfet is grateful to work, live, and cultivate knowledge on the traditional territory of the Syilx Okanagan people.

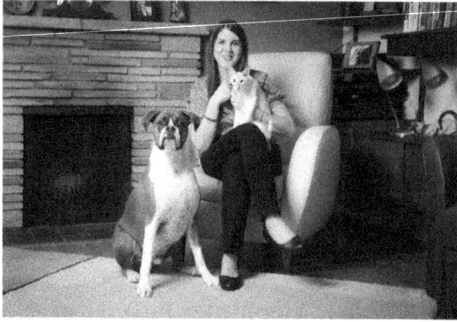

Christine Yvette Tardif-Williams, PhD, is a professor in the Department of Child and Youth Studies at Brock University. Her research adopts both basic and applied approaches and is informed by the interdisciplinary fields of child and youth studies and human-animal interactions. Her research focuses more broadly on how close bonds between humans and animals shape the social and emotional lives of children and youth. Specifically, her research examines human-animal interactions, children's interactions with animals (within family, school, and virtual contexts), and various aspects of parent-child relationships. Her research on children's and dog handlers' experiences with animals and therapy dogs in a variety of contexts has been published in *Anthrozoös*, *Society and Animals*, *Human-Animal Interactions*, and *Pet Behavior Science*. She is the co-author of a recently published book titled *Virtual Human-Animal Interactions: Supporting Learning, Social Connections and Well-Being* (Tardif-Williams & Binfet, 2023; Routledge).

Dr. Tardif-Williams is grateful to work, live, and cultivate knowledge on the traditional territory of the Haudenosaunee and Anishinaabe peoples.

Meet the Authors

Introduction

One

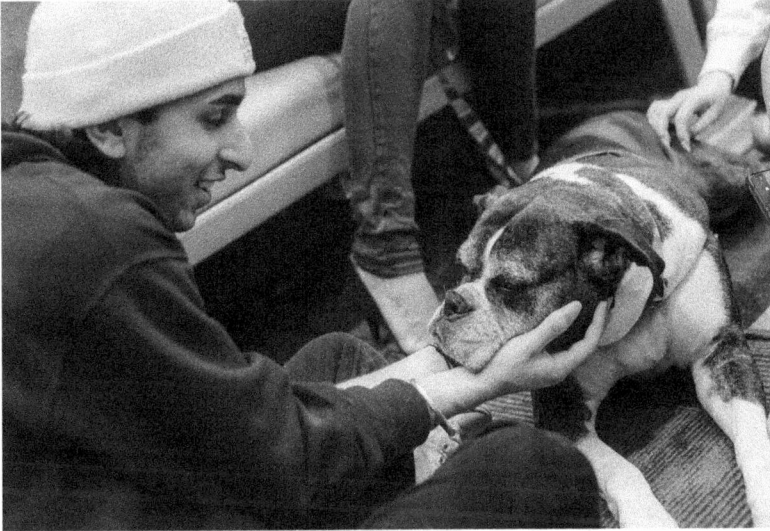

Figure 1.1 An undergraduate student cups the face of therapy dog Maya, a Boxer
Source: F. L. L. Green Photography; used with permission

1 Introduction

DOI: 10.4324/9781032639284-1

Simultaneously Over- and Underwhelmed

At her local dog park, Susan heard about a therapy dog program operating at a nearby college that ran stress reduction sessions for students during exam periods. As she'd recently retired, Susan had time to volunteer. Added to this, her six-year-old Golden Retriever Ollie loved people. She and Ollie easily passed the certification process and found themselves assigned to a Friday evening session along with three other dog-handler teams. Upon arrival, it was clear that the demand for access to the dogs surpassed the capacity to support the line of students snaking around the building. To Susan's surprise, there was no program organizer onsite and the dog handlers were left to set up their stations, whilst a student volunteer tried to corral and contain the excited students waiting in line. Students were given only five minutes to visit one of the dog-handler teams, and Susan did her best to connect with the students who came to her station. Susan noticed no water was made available and she hadn't thought to bring a bowl with her. After 90 minutes, the session was terminated despite the long line of students remaining. Some of the students even followed Susan and Ollie to the parking lot, so desperate were they to have even a brief opportunity to interact with Ollie. Susan left the campus feeling like she'd just participated in some sort of high-speed therapy dog factory where student visitors were shuffled through her station with little opportunity to share information about Ollie or, more importantly, strategies around how best to interact with him. Upon arriving home, Susan was exhausted and Ollie drank profusely. Before retiring for the night, Susan sent an email to the director of the therapy dog program indicating she was happy to volunteer but not for student sessions during exam periods (Figure 1.1).

QUESTIONS FOR REFLECTION AND DISCUSSION

1. How should canine-assisted interventions (CAIs) be structured? Is guidance or supervision by program personnel required? If so, what is their role?

2. For how long should visits be scheduled?

3. How many visitors should a dog-handler team support during a session? How might the number of visitors to a dog-handler station impact the therapy dog?

4. Does a dog handler have a responsibility to educate visitors about how to interact with a therapy dog? If so, what should be shared?

5. To optimize therapy dog welfare, what provisions are required for dogs within a session?

6. What is the responsibility of program personnel to support volunteer dog-handler teams?

Like you, we share a passion for therapy dogs. We've seen the good work they can do in supporting clients ranging from college students seeking to reduce their stress, to school children seeking to bolster their reading skills in an after-school program at a local library, and offering social and emotional support to children at summer camp, lonely seniors in a retirement care facility, and stressed law enforcement officers in a busy urban detachment. We're keen to understand how to optimize interactions between visitors to a CAI so that animal and human welfare is prioritized and safeguarded. What follows in this book is an exploration and examination of therapy dog-handler team welfare. We acknowledge upfront that we have chosen to primarily focus on the welfare of therapy dogs but recognize that the dog-handler team works in a collaborative synergy and that the collective welfare of the dog-handler team must be considered as handlers are key agents overseeing, guiding, and optimizing dog welfare. In effect, dog handlers are responsible for implementing welfare measures that support and optimize the work that therapy dogs do within sessions.

The overarching aims of our book are threefold: First, to review the extant literature on therapy dog welfare and dog welfare more broadly; second, to examine handler welfare within the context of CAIs; and third, to offer applied insights and recommendations to optimize the dog-handler team welfare whilst working in sessions to support human well-being. This chapter will elucidate key terminology as it pertains to dog-handler teams and the work they undertake to support human well-being, and define welfare within the broader context of human-animal interactions (HAIs) and more specifically within the context of CAIs. We'll conclude the chapter by establishing why safeguarding and optimizing dog-handler team welfare is important – concepts we'll revisit throughout the book.

CLARIFYING TERMINOLOGY

It's important at the outset to define and differentiate key terminology used throughout our book. This will help equip readers as they navigate their way through empirical findings and practical applied strategies. The field of HAI is replete with acronyms (saturated even some might argue; Green et al., 2024; Johnson Binder et al., 2024), and we've done our best to streamline key terminology pertinent to dog-handler team welfare (see Table 1.1).

CAIS, ANIMAL VISITATION PROGRAMS, AND ANIMAL-ASSISTED PROGRAMS

Table 1.1 provides an overview of common terminology used by researchers and practitioners working under the broad umbrella of

Table 1.1 Overview of Key Terminology Used Throughout Our Book

Terminology and Acronym	Definition
Human-animal interactions (HAIs)	"…A broad term that refers to any manner of relationship or behavior between people and animal(s)" (American Veterinary Medical Association, 2024b)
Human-animal bond (HAB)	"The human-animal bond is a mutually beneficial relationship between people and animals. It's influenced by behaviors essential to the mental, physical, and social health and wellbeing of both." (American Veterinary Medical Association, 2024a) "Mutually beneficial emotional, psychological and physical interactions that lead to a relationship that supports the health and well-being of both humans and animals." (Animal-Assisted Intervention International, 2021)
Animal-assisted interventions (AAIs)	"An Animal Assisted Intervention is a goal oriented and structured intervention that intentionally includes or incorporates animals in health, education, and human services (e.g., social work) for the purpose of therapeutic gains in humans." (IAHAIO, 2018)

Terminology and Acronym	Definition
Animal-assisted activities (AAAs)	"AAA is a planned and goal oriented informal interaction and visitation conducted by the human-animal team for motivational, educational, and recreational purposes." (IAHAIO, 2018)
Canine-assisted interventions (CAIs)	"The bringing together of credentialed CAI teams and members of the public in a specified setting with the purpose of enhancing human well-being. May be delivered individually with one CAI team and one client or group administered with several CAI teams supporting multiple clients." (Binfet & Hartwig, 2020, p. 10)
Dog-handler team	"A term to describe a therapy dog and handler or practitioner who work collaboratively within CAIs as volunteers for an organization or as professional practitioners." (Binfet & Hartwig, 2020, p. 10)
Therapy dogs	"Therapy dogs are trained to provide comfort and affection to people other than their handlers or owners. That could mean visiting a variety of places where people need love and affection, such as hospitals, schools, hospices, nursing homes, disaster areas, and more." (Alliance of Therapy Dogs, 2022, para. 2) "A dog assessed for behavior, skills, and disposition who works under the guidance of a handler or practitioner and who participates in interactions to support the social, emotional, and/or physical development of clients." (Binfet & Hartwig, 2020, p. 10) "It should also be noted that therapy animals are pets who have been evaluated on their ability to safely interact with a wide range of populations. They differ from service animals and from emotional support animals in that their role is to provide interactions to people other than their handlers in their working role." (Pet Partners, 2021 as cited in Fine & Chastain Griffin, 2022)
Client (for CAI specifically)	"An individual in a community or professional setting who interacts with a CAI team in an effort to promote wellness." (Binfet & Hartwig, 2020, p. 10)
Program coordinator	A volunteer or paid position who organizes and oversees all aspects of programming involving dog-handler teams.

HAI, yet additional discussion of three key and sometimes overlapping terms is warranted. CAIs are defined as a purposeful intervention whose aim is to provide opportunities for human participants to spend time and interact with therapy dogs to bolster their well-being (e.g., happiness, interpersonal connections) and reduce their ill-being (e.g., stress, loneliness, homesickness; Binfet, 2023). CAIs are often introduced as part of experimental studies whose aim is to ascertain pre-to-post-interaction changes experienced by participants as measured in various outcome variables (and then often compared to findings from control participants). Parallel terms such as *Animal-Assisted Programs* (AAPs; Haggerty & Mueller, 2017) and *Animal Visitation Programs* (AVPs; Carr & Pendry, 2024) are also evident in the literature and reflect researcher preference. Recent research on the prevalence of terminology and their corresponding acronyms by Green and colleagues (2024) identified the field of HAI as particularly saturated with new terminology and acronyms, and moreover, once introduced, there is often little uptake of newly introduced terms by others publishing HAI-related research. These researchers also found the prevalence of duplicating yet distinct terminology to describe similar interventions or aspects of HAI and animal-assisted intervention (AAI; e.g., canine-assisted therapy and canine therapy).

It merits noting that, in comparison with the term *CAIs*, AAPs and AVPs both suggest that animals other than dogs may be involved in the HAI. That is, the term *CAI* clearly indicates for readers that the study results or the topic at hand explicitly incorporates therapy dogs and no other animals who may participate in HAIs. For the purposes of our book and, as our book is devoted to deeply understanding welfare issues in working therapy dog-handler teams, we will employ the term *CAI* to refer to interventions in which human participants interact with a dog-handler team with the intent of boosting well-being and reducing ill-being. We'll revisit this distinction again in Chapter 2 when providing a retrospective of the field of CAIs.

THE PROLIFIC GROWTH OF THE FIELD OF HAIS

HAI researchers have documented the rapid rise in HAI research as reflected by both the number of publications and their corresponding citations. Recent research by Rodriguez and colleagues (2023; see Figure 1.2) chronicled this growth.

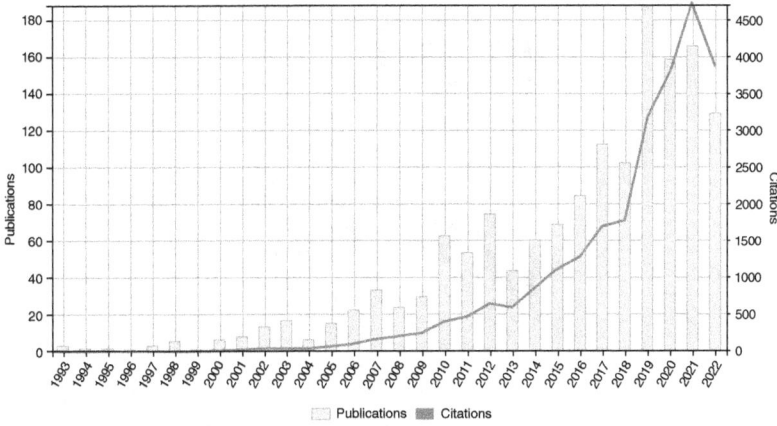

Figure 1.2 Illustration of the growth of AAIs

Source: Human-Animal Interactions; used with permission

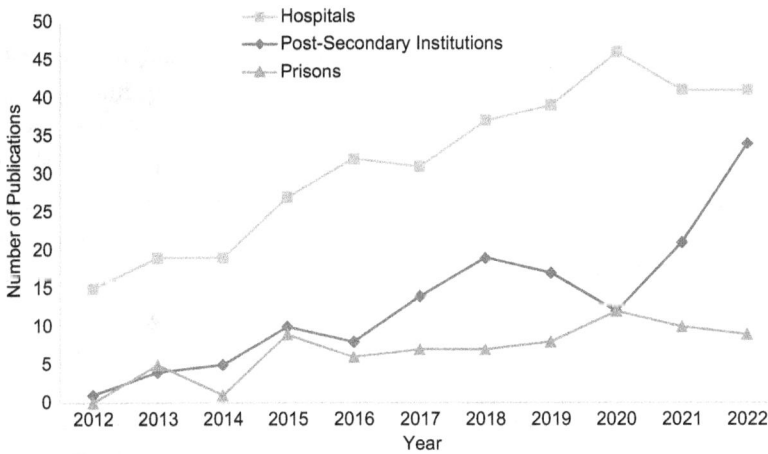

Figure 1.3 Publication trends of AAIs

Source: Fine et al., 2025; used with permission

Mirroring this growth trajectory, a recent scan by Binfet et al. (2025) examined the number of publications extolling findings from CAIs administered in college, prison, and hospital settings (see Figure 1.3). In concert with Figure 1.2, in Figure 1.3 we see exponential growth in the research interest in, and the number of subsequent publications by researchers examining the effects of AAIs on human well-being in three popular contexts for HAI research.

Publication Trends of AAIs in Post-Secondary Institutions, Hospitals, and Correctional Facilities from 2012–2023

Note. see the following URL or QR code for search protocol and analyses:

https://bit.ly/OSF_AAI_LitMap.

Also reflecting both the proliferation of publications of research conducted in HAI and AAI and the corresponding academic interest in this research are review publications synthesizing findings as reported in meta-analyses, systematic reviews, and scoping reviews (see Table 1.2 for illustrations of recent review publications). The sheer volume of recent reviews reflects the depth of rich empirical work being done in the fields of HAI and AAI – that is, one cannot synthesize findings across studies unless there are studies to compare and contrast. Table 1.2 attests to the depth of HAI (and CAI) publications.

Table 1.2 Illustrations of Recent Review Papers in HAI and CAI

Title	Number of Publications Examined	Authors
Examining evidence for a relationship between human-animal interactions and common mental disorders during the COVID-19 pandemic: A systematic literature review.	1,721 articles screened 21 publications included in review	Barr et al. (2024).
Animal-assisted interventions in universities: A scoping review of implementation and associated outcomes.	1,467 articles screened 47 publications included in review	Cooke et al. (2022).

Title	Number of Publications Examined	Authors
How to measure human-dog interaction in dog-assisted interventions? A scoping review.	412 articles screen 70 publications included in review	De Santis et al. (2024)
A systematic review of research on pet ownership and animal interactions among older adults.	24,263 articles screened 145 publications included in review	Gee and Mueller (2019)
Can canine-assisted interventions affect the social behaviours of children on the Autism Spectrum? A systematic review.	3,752 articles screened 13 publications included in review	Hill et al. (2019)
Dog-assisted interventions and outcomes for older adults in residential long-term care facilities: A systematic review and meta-analysis.	5,773 articles screened 43 publications included in review	Jain et al. (2020).
Examining human-animal interactions and their effect on multidimensional frailty in later life: A scoping review.	3,118 articles screened 4 publications included in review	Taeckens et al. (2023).
Specific and non-specific factors of animal-assisted interventions considered in research: A systematic review.	2,001 articles screened and 172 publications included in review	Wagner et al. (2022)
Human-animal interactions in disaster settings: A systematic review	334 articles screened 94 publications included in review	Wu et al. (2023)

DEFINING WELFARE IN THE CONTEXT OF CAIS

In HAI research, the animal is a quiet partner, useful only for the effect their presence has on the person, and rarely considered in and of themselves.

(Horowitz, 2021, p. 1)

Horowitz's observation above offers a utilitarian interpretation of how animals might be viewed and situated within the context of HAI research. Whilst this view may well characterize HAI research of the past, as researchers conducting CAI studies, we increasingly see animal welfare at the forefront of interventions and research protocols. In fact, we've become advocates for repositioning therapy dogs as

Therapy dog welfare and signs of distress were monitored during each session by a trained research assistant, familiar with the therapy dogs. Therapy dogs were provided with a 15-minute opportunity to settle prior to the session commencing, during which the research assistant would monitor their body language and behavior. When the dogs were present on camera, they were seated on the floor or a large sofa with their handler, much like they would be at home. When dogs were not present in the video, they were provided with a comfortable spot to rest close to their handler (but out of camera view) and were under the supervision of a volunteer with whom they were familiar. The total involvement of the dogs was a maximum of 15 minutes in front of the camera and one-hour in total on-location. In addition, dogs were only permitted to be involved in sessions twice per week and not on consecutive days; typically, they were involved only once per week. If a dog (or handler) showed any signs of distress during a filming or Zoom session, they were sent home; this did not occur in this study and no incidents of canine distress were reported.

Figure 1.4 Description of canine welfare in published research
Source: Binfet et al., 2022a in *Anthrozoös*; used with permission

partners in research, and our hope is this book situates dog welfare front and centre in applied programming, research interventions, and publications – as a means of honouring and celebrating the good work that dog-handler teams do to support human well-being. To illustrate this, take, for example, our description of canine welfare within a recent publication assessing the effects of virtual canine comfort modules on undergraduate students' stress (Binfet et al., 2022a, p. 816; see Figure 1.4).

DEFINING THERAPY DOG WELFARE

As a starting point, it's important to define welfare within the context of CAIs as our understanding of welfare here informs the policies and practices recommended throughout our book. We'll explore and define more precisely the concept of therapy dog welfare in Chapter 3, but as initial definitions of welfare, we lean on prior definitions provided by the nascent work of Broom (1986, p. 524) who defined animal welfare as "the state of an animal as regards its attempts to cope with its environment" and the work of Ng and colleagues (2015, p. 359) who build on Broom's definition and capture key elements comprising animal welfare.

Very good welfare and well-being status is characterized by a state in which an animal is free from distress most of the time, is in good

physical health, exhibits a substantial range of species-specific
behaviors, and is able to cope effectively with environmental stimuli.

(Hetts et al., 1992; Novak & Drewsen, 1989).

Absent from this definition, and a topic we'll revisit and explore in Chapters 3 and 5, is the concept of consent and the importance of obtaining consent from an animal prior to initiating interaction. Inherent in both Broom's and Ng et al.,'s definitions is the recognition that environmental stimuli hold potential to compromise animal welfare. An examination of the anticipated and unanticipated environmental stimuli therapy dogs face in CAIs is discussed in Chapters 3 and 5.

RECOGNIZING HOMOGENEITY AND VARIABILITY IN CAIS

CAIs vary in nearly every way; their only common trait is the involvement of dogs to respond to human need.

(Meers et al., 2022, p. 1)

CAIs draw researchers and practitioners from varied fields and disciplines. In this regard and given their varied background training, they bring diverse perspectives of welfare. Across varied CAI publications, we see researchers with backgrounds in *Education*, *Child and Youth Studies*, *Anthrozoology*, *Psychology*, *Sociology*, *Nursing*, and *Occupational Therapy*, among other disciplines. Certainly, one hope for our book is that increased discussion and a greater consensus around the conceptualization and actualization of welfare practices can result.

In Chapter 2, we'll examine more closely the effects of CAIs on various dimensions of human well-being; however, it's important to recognize the range of interventions researchers implement as part of CAIs. There is enormous variability in the screening, selection, and training of dog-handler teams, in the duration of the intervention itself, in the ratio of clients to therapy dogs within a session, in the total number of sessions offered, in the monitoring and safeguarding of canine welfare, and in researchers' recognition that the quality (or rigour) of the CAI itself plays a predominant role in intervention efficacy. Next, we examine key factors that comprise a CAI.

Despite the claims above proclaiming there is great variability in CAIs, there remains one element or factor that is largely homogenous – the handlers themselves. At the outset of this chapter, we defined the dog-handler team as "A term to describe a therapy dog and handler or practitioner who work collaboratively within CAIs as volunteers for an organization or as professional practitioners" (Binfet & Hartwig, 2020, p. 10). There is but scant published research on handlers and the role they play in either applied programming or research.

We can glean from descriptions reported as part of published studies that, by and large, volunteer dog handlers appear to be women typically ranging in age from 40 to 60 years (Rousseau et al., 2020). Though infrequently reported, many, we suspect, are retired and seeking to contribute in meaningful ways to their community by sharing their love for their dog. In one of the few published studies on volunteer handlers, Rousseau and colleagues (2020) surveyed 60 dog handlers to explore and understand their experiences participating in an on-campus CAI. Their findings revealed a portrait of volunteer dog handlers comprised of predominantly female (87%), almost entirely White (97%), and with 77% having a college degree. Their mean age was 42 years (SD = 12.96), and handlers in this study had, on average, 7.5 years of prior therapy dog volunteer experience. It merits noting too that the volunteers in this study spent almost eight hours per semester volunteering within the context of CAIs.

In a second study examining the motivations of handlers volunteering with Pet Partners, a large US agency promoting, supporting, and overseeing HAI programming, Kirnan et al. (2024) provided a profile of volunteer handlers (N = 748) as predominantly female (upwards of 87%), predominantly White (91%), and with a mean age of 61 years (range = 15–86). Collectively, the studies by Rousseau et al. (2020) and Kirnan and colleagues (2024) inform our understanding of who is inclined to volunteer as a dog handler in CAIs.

Beyond the immediate realm of CAIs yet field-adjacent as their work involves therapy dogs is recent research by Eaton-Stull and colleagues (2023) who identify the characteristics of dogs and handlers working in animal-assisted crisis response (AACR). These dog-handler teams provide comfort and support to individuals who experience disasters and crises across the globe. Considering the work they undertake, it's not surprising that AACR dog-handler teams or crisis-response teams require advanced training and must meet AACR national standards (see Eaton-Stull et al., 2010 here). Consider, for a moment, just what is asked of these dogs and their handlers – to fly on short notice to disaster sites and provide comfort and support to strangers in contexts full of confusion, strife, struggle, and heightened emotions. In their survey of 99 AACR handlers, these researchers identified findings consistent with the findings reported above characterizing handlers. Notably, handlers were predominantly women (88%), ranged in age from 61 to 70 years, almost half were retired, and, on average, handlers had 5.7 years prior experience in AACR. A point raised by these authors, and perhaps the motivation underlying their study, is that accessing handlers for this specialized work is especially challenging. In Chapter 3, we'll examine the complexities of accessing volunteer CAI dog-handler teams.

Understanding the characteristics of handlers is important as handlers are a key factor overseeing their dog's welfare and a key agent contributing to the efficacy of the CAI itself. An excerpt from one of our recent publications on the effects of a virtual CAI illustrates how both handlers and therapy dogs might be described as part of a study (see Figure 1.5). Positioning the handlers and therapy dogs as central participants in a study serves to honour their contribution to empirical investigations and helps describe their experience as part of the intervention.

Canine Handlers

Community volunteer canine handlers and their therapy canines were drawn from a larger pool of 55 certified handlers and canines involved in the university's B.A.R.K. canine therapy program. Six volunteer handlers participated in this study (100% female, 100% Caucasian, M_{age} = 49.4 years, SD = 11.3, range = 37–67 years, M prior canine therapy experience = 5.01 years, SD = 3.40).

Therapy Canines

Chosen from the larger pool of 56 therapy dogs working in the B.A.R.K. program, six therapy canines participated in this study (66% female, M_{age} = 6.39 years, SD = 2.25, range = 4–10 years, prior canine therapy experience = 4.01 years, SD = 2.54). Participating canines included: 1 Golden Retriever, 1 Labrador, 1 Norwegian Elkhund, and 3 mixed breeds (including a Border Collie cross, Great Dane/Labrador mix and Golden/Bernese Mountain Dog Mix).

Figure 1.5 Illustrations of handler and therapy dog descriptions

Source: Binfet et al. (2022a) in *Anthrozoös;* used with permission

Embedded within the demographic description of the handlers above, we see their average prior experience reported in years (Binfet et al., 2022a). This can be helpful in recognizing that the intervention itself was delivered by experienced or veteran handlers – handlers who have ample prior volunteer experience in delivering CAIs. It merits noting that not all researchers seek this experience but rather that prior experience could be a controlled variable. In Clark and colleagues' (2020) study assessing handler cortisol within the context of a hospital setting, prior experience as a handler was not sought. These researchers describe:

> A therapy dog team consists of a dog and a handler who have passed a therapy dog test and are considered a registered team. All teams that applied to the Caring Canines program at Mayo Clinic Rochester that had not volunteered with another dog or in another setting were asked to participate in the study. Handlers who had visited with other dogs were excluded, and dogs who had visited anywhere else were excluded as well. The team had to be a new team with no experience at Mayo Clinic, Rochester, MN, where all visits took place.
>
> (Clark et al., 2020, p. 2)

We thus see ample variability in the prior experience of handlers as they participate in studies assessing the effects of CAIs on human well-being. Recall Susan, the handler in our opening scenario, who was a new handler who found herself overwhelmed in an on-campus CAI. With no support from a program coordinator and with little applied experience herself to lean on, Susan and her dog Ollie were overwhelmed by the busy and haphazard nature of the programming they'd been asked to support.

Handler prior experience might typically be considered an asset adding value to the intervention. That is, the more seasoned the handler, the stronger the implementation fidelity of the intervention (i.e., that the intervention was delivered as intended). To support or guide handlers, some researchers ask handlers to follow a script (see Appendix 1.1 for an example). Such was the case for a recent study exploring the role of touch in CAIs that asked handlers to adhere to a guideline comprised of questions they might ask participants (Binfet et al., 2022b). This was done to standardize the experience of participants across handlers and, in turn, help minimize confounding variables such as handler personality or ability to engage participants as part of the intervention. Returning to our opening scenario, as a new handler with little training and no prior experience, Susan would be ill-equipped to participate in a CAI requiring handlers to follow specific protocols to engage participants. Through no fault of her own, including Susan in a CAI to assess the effects of a CAI on various outcome variables could compromise the quality of the intervention itself and/or the overall rigour of the study.

HONOURING THE THERAPY DOG'S EXPERIENCE

There is a risk that dogs may be viewed solely as tools to provide emotional or therapeutic support rather than as individuals with their own needs and desires.

(McDowall et al., 2023, p. 1)

The above excerpt from researchers McDowall and colleagues (2023) highlights the importance of recognizing the nuanced contribution of therapy dogs and their positioning within CAIs. Echoing Horowitz's (2021) earlier description of therapy dogs as quiet partners, rarely considered, here we see researchers recognize the individuality of, and needs of, the therapy dog participating in interventions to bolster human well-being.

Just as the training and experience of handlers impacts their ability to participate in CAIs, the experience of therapy dogs too impacts their participation in CAIs. Increasingly, researchers are reporting, in detail, the characteristics of the therapy dogs participating in CAIs. Take, for example, our description above from one of our studies examining the role of therapy dogs in eliciting well-being outcomes in under-graduate students within a virtual context (Binfet et al., 2022a). This detailed description is key to the study as the dogs played a pivotal role in the intervention and their ability to demonstrate the skills required of therapy dogs enhances (or detracts from) the intervention itself. Recent research by Carr and Pendry (2024, p. 61) provides a description of the therapy dogs who participated in their study as well as reference to dog-handler teams (Figure 1.6).

Human–Dog Teams

Human–dog teams were trained, evaluated, and registered members of Palouse Paws, a local regional community partner of the Pet Partners national organization (Pet Partners, 2019). Teams (n = 29) consisted of 48% male dogs (100% neutered), 48% female dogs (71% spayed; 29% intact), and 4% unspecified status. Dogs ranged in age from 7 months to 13.5 years and averaged 4 years 7 months in age. Dogs were most commonly retrievers (Labrador = 21%; Golden = 14% Golden-Labrador = 3%), followed by mixed breeds (21%) and other breeds (e.g., Great Dane, Shetland Sheepdog, Pitbull). On average, dogs participated in 2.5 h of community visits (libraries, schools, hospital, etc.) per week (range: 1–13 h per week) with Palouse Paws. Most handlers were middle-aged women (76%; M_{age} = 52.3 years; min = 22, max = 73) and had on average three years of volunteer experience, which ranged from "first timer[s]" to eight-year veterans. Fifteen teams were familiar with the program area having volunteered as a part of a prior study. Handlers and dogs were invited to attend an orientation meeting prior to the start of the program during which the study procedures and expectations were explained in detail.

Figure 1.6 Description of therapy dogs participating in research
Source: Carr & Pendry, 2024 in *Anthrozoös*; used with permission

WELFARE IMPLICATIONS FOR CAI RESEARCH

It seems logical that good welfare not only benefits the animal but also has a positive impact on the overall efficacy of the entire interaction.

(Fine & Chastain Griffin, 2022, p. 12)

As the field of HAI advances and the delivery of interventions involving therapy dogs become more fully understood and sophisticated, it is important to recognize that dog-handler team welfare is an essential and important factor determining the quality of the intervention itself. In our opening scenario, Susan, a volunteer dog handler, and her therapy dog Ollie found themselves in a fast-paced environment that Susan described as a "high-speed therapy dog factory." Not only was the intervention itself brief, but the constant turnover of clients combined with their heightened excitement created less-than-optimal conditions for interactions and ultimately compromised the potency of the CAI. Moving beyond a mere discussion of whether welfare considerations are present or absent, it's important to assess the quality of the welfare measures implemented for any given CAI.

OVERVIEW OF FORTHCOMING CHAPTERS

In this chapter, we shared the overarching aims of our book, defined welfare within the context of working therapy dogs and their handlers, and provided a preliminary overview of the ways of safeguarding dog-handler team welfare to optimize the good work that these teams undertake in supporting varied human clients. In the chapter that follows next, we examine the history of CAIs. Here we look at the origins of programs and interventions that provide opportunities for varied members of the public to interact with therapy dogs. In Chapter 3, we explore, in depth, the welfare of dog-handler teams. Here we examine the relationship between handlers and dogs and how welfare can enhance or compromise the interplay between handlers and dogs. In Chapter 4, and from a proactive perspective, we examine the factors known to predict a dog-handler's team ability to work effectively within CAIs – that is, what contributes to a team working optimally? In Chapter 5, we explore the factors that both hinder and compromise a team's ability to work in CAIs as well as factors that characterize a successful dog-handler team. Next, in Chapter 6, we explore welfare across varied contexts including post-secondary, public school, hospital, and correctional facilities that might see dog handlers introduced to support client well-being. In Chapter 7, we identify policies and procedures that safeguard welfare and provide rationales undergirding their implementation. In our concluding chapter, Chapter 8, we revisit the key concepts and arguments identified throughout the book and cast an eye to the future, situating CAIs in under-researched contexts and raising welfare considerations therein.

REFERENCES

Alliance of Therapy Dogs. (2022, May 27). *What do therapy dogs actually do?* https://www.therapydogs.com/what-do-therapy-dogs-actually-do/

American Veterinary Medical Association. (2024a). *Human-animal bond.* https://www.avma.org/resources-tools/one-health/human-animal-bond

American Veterinary Medical Association. (2024b). *Human-animal interaction and the human-animal bond.* https://www.avma.org/resources-tools/avma-policies/human-animal-interaction-and-human-animal-bond#:~:text=Human%2Danimal%20 interaction%20a%20broad,%2C%20community%2C%20or%20societal%20 contexts

Animal Assisted Intervention International (2021). Glossary of terms. Retrieved July 10, 2014 from https://aai-int.org/aai/glossary-of-terms/

Barr, H. K., Guggenbickler, A. M., Hoch, J. S., & Dewa, C. S. (2024). Examining evidence for a relationship between human-animal interactions and common mental disorders during the COVID-19 pandemic: A systematic review. *Frontiers in Health Services, 4,* 1321293. https://doi.org/10.3389/frhs.2024.1321293

Binfet, J. T. (2023). Canine-assisted interventions: Insights from the B.A.R.K. program and future research directions. In J. Stevens (Ed.), *Canine cognition and the human bond* (pp. 117–134). Springer.

Binfet, J. T., Green, F. L. L., & Draper, Z. A. (2022b). The importance of client-canine contact in canine-assisted interventions: A randomized controlled trial. *Anthrozoös*, 35(1), 1–22. https://doi.org/10.1080/08927936.2021.1944558

Binfet, J.T. & Hartwig, E.K. (2020). *Canine-assisted interventions: A comprehensive guide to credentialing therapy dog teams.* Routledge.

Binfet, J.T., Rousseau, C. X., & Green, F. L. L. (2025). Animal-assisted interventions in specialized settings: Findings, complexities, and considerations in post-secondary, hospital, and correctional contexts. In Fine, A. H., Mueller, M. K., Ng, Z., Griffin, T. C., & Tedeschi, P. (Eds.), *Handbook on animal-assisted therapy* (6th ed.). Elsevier.

Binfet, J.T., Tardif-Williams, C., Draper, Z. A., Green, F. L. L., Singal, A., Rousseau, C. X., & Roma, R. (2022a). Virtual canine comfort: A randomized controlled trial of the effects of a canine-assisted intervention supporting undergraduate wellbeing. *Anthrozoös*, 35(6), 809–832. https://doi: 10.1080/08927936.2022.2062866

Broom, D. (1986). Indicators of poor welfare. Protecting dog welfare safeguards human welfare. *British Veterinary Journal*, 142, 524–526. https://doi.org/10.1016/0007-1935(86)90109-0

Carr, A. M. & Pendry, P. (2024). Assessing attendance frequency and duration at a drop-in animal visitation program among first-semester university students separated from their pets. *Anthrozoös*, 37(1), 55–74. Https://doi.org/10.1080/08927936.2023.2261281

Clark, S. D., Smidt, J. M., & Bauer, B. A. (2020). Therapy dogs' and handlers' behavior and salivary cortisol during initial visits in a complex medical institution: A pilot study. *Frontiers in Veterinary Science*, 7, 564201. Https://doi.org/10.3389/fvets.2020.564201

Cooke, E., Henderson-Wilson, C., Warner, E., & LaMontagne, A. (2022). Animal-assisted interventions in universities: A scoping review of implementation and associated outcomes. *Health Promotion International*, 38(3), daac001. https://doi.org/10.1093/heapro/daac001

De Santis, M., Filugelli, L., Mair, A., Normando, S., Mutinelli, F., & Contalbrigo, L. (2024). How to measure human-dog interaction in dog assisted interventions? A scoping review. *Animals*, 14(3). https://doi.org/10.3390/ani14030410

Eaton-Stull, Y. M., Ehlers, C., Ganse, D., Lothrop, G., & Rideout, A. (2010). Animal assisted crisis response national standards. *National Standards Committee for Animal-Assisted Crisis Response*, 1-13. Available at: https://www.hopeaacr.org/wpcontent/uploads/2010/03/AACRNationalStandards7Mar10.pdf.

Eaton-Stull, Y. M., Jaffe, B., Scott, K., & Shiller, M. (2023). Animal-assisted crisis response: Characteristics of canine handlers and their canine partners. *Human-Animal Interactions*, 11(1), https://doi.org/10.1079/hai.2023.0033

Fine, A. H. & Chastain Griffin, T. (2022). Protecting animal welfare in animal-assisted intervention: Our ethical obligation. *Seminars in Speech and Language*, 43, (1), 8–23. Https://doi.org/10.1055/s-0041-1742099

Fine, A. H., Mueller, M. K., Ng, Z., Griffin, T. C., & Tedeschi, P. (2025). *Handbook on animal-assisted therapy* (6th ed.). Elsevier.

Gee, N. R. & Mueller, M. K. (2019). A systematic review of research on pet ownership and animal interactions among older adults. *Anthrozoös, 32*(2), 183–307. https://doi.org/10.1080/08927936.2019.1569903

Green, F. L. L., Dahlman, M., Lomness, A., & Binfet, J. T. (2024). For the love of acronyms: An analysis of terminology and acronyms used in AAI research. *Human-Animal Interactions, 12* (1), https://doi.org/10.1079/hai.2024.0024

Haggerty, J. M., & Mueller, M. K. (2017). Animal-assisted stress reduction programs in higher education. *Innovation in Higher Education, 42*, 379–389. https://doi.org/10.1007/s10755-017-9392-0.

Hetts, S., Clark, J. D., Arnold, C. E., & Mateo, J. M. (1992). Influence of housing conditions on beagle behaviour. *Applied Animal Behavior Science, 34*, 137–155.

Hill, J., Ziviani, J., Driscoll, C., & Cawdell-Smith, J. (2019). Can canine-assisted interventions affect the social behaviours of children on the autism spectrum? A systematic review. *Review Journal of Autism and Developmental Disorders, 6*, 13–25. https://doi.org/10.1007/s40489-018-0151-7

Horowitz, A. (2021). Consider the "Dog" in dog-human interaction. *Frontiers in Veterinary Science, 8*, 642821. Https://doi.org/10.3389/fvets.2021.642821

International Association of Human-Animal Interaction Organizations. (2018). *The IAHAIO definitions for animal assisted intervention and guidelines for wellness of animals involved in AAI* [White paper]. IAHAIO. https://iahaio.org/best-practice/white-paper-on-animal-assisted-interventions/

Jain, B., Syed, S., Hafford-Letchfield, T., & O'Farrell-Pearce, S. (2020). Dog-assisted interventions and outcomes for older adults in residential long-term care facilities: A systematic review and meta-analysis. *International Journal of Older People Nursing, 15*(3), e12320. https://doi.org/10.1111/opn.12320

Johnson Binder, A., Parish-Plass, N., Kirby M., Winkle, M., Plesa Skwerer, D., . . . Winjen, B. (2024). Recommendations for uniform terminology in animal-assisted services (AAS). *Human-Animal Interactions, 12*(1). https://docs.lib.purdue.edu/cgi/viewcontent.cgi?article=1144&context=paij

Kirnan, J., Ciarrocca, A., & Malloy, M. (2024). "My dog needs a job": Identifying the motivations of therapy animal volunteers. *People and Animals: The International Journal of Research and Practice, 7*(1), Article 6. https://docs.lib.purdue.edu/paij/vol7/iss1/6

McDowall, S., Hazel, S. J., Cobb, M., & Hamilton-Bruce, A. (2023). Understanding the role of therapy dogs in human health promotion. *International Journal of Environmental Research and Public Health, 20*, 5801. Https://doi.org/10.3390/ijerph20105801

Meers, L. L., Contalbrigo, L., Samuels, W. E., Duarte-Gan, C., Berckmans, D., . . . Normando, S. (2022). Canine-assisted interventions and the relevance of welfare assessments for human health, and transmission of zoonosis: A literature review. *Frontiers in Veterinary Science, 9*, e899889. Https://doi.org/10.3389/fvets.2022.899889

Ng, Z., Albright, J., Fine, A. H., & Peralta, J. (2015). Our ethical and moral responsibility: Ensuring the welfare of therapy animals. In A. Fine (Ed.), *Handbook on animal-assisted therapy* (4th ed., pp. 357–376). Elsevier.

Novak, M. A., & Drewsen, K. H. (1989). Enriching the lives of captive primates: Issues and problems. In E. F. Segal (Ed.), *Housing, care, and psychological wellbeing of captive and laboratory primates* (pp. 161–185). Noyes.

Pet Partners (2021). *Terminology*. https://petpartners.org/publications/glossary/

Rodriguez, K. E., Green, F. L. L., Binfet, J. T., Townsend, L., & Gee, N. (2023). Complexities and considerations in conducting animal-assisted intervention research: A discussion of randomized controlled trials. *Human–Animal Interactions.* https://doi.org/10.1079/hai.2023.0004

Rousseau, C. X., Binfet, J. T., Green, F. L. L., Tardif-Williams, C. Y., Draper, Z. A., & Maynard, A. (2020). Up the leash: Exploring canine handlers' perceptions of volunteering in canine-assisted interventions. *Pet Behaviour Science, 10,* 15–35. https://doi.org/10.21071/pbs.vi10.12598

Taeckens, A., Corcoran, M., Wang, K., & Morris, K. N. (2023). Examining human-animal interactions and their effect on multidimensional frailty in later life: A scoping review. *Frontiers in Public Health, 21*(11), 1214127. https://doi.org/10.3389/fpubh.2023.1214127

Wagner, C., Grob, C., & Hediger, K. (2022). Specific and non-specific factors of animal-assisted interventions considered in research: A systematic review. *Frontiers in Psychology, 13,* e931347. https://doi.org/10.3389/fpsyg.2022.931347

Wu, H., Heyland, L. K., Yung, M., & Schneider, M. (2023). Human-animal interactions in disaster settings: A systematic review. *International Journal of Disaster Risk Science, 14,* 369–381. https://doi.org/10.1007/s13753-023-00496-9

APPENDIX 1.1

Example Guidelines for Handlers from Binfet et al. (2022a)

SEMISTRUCTURED QUESTION GUIDE FOR HANDLERS

This series of questions are designed to be a guide to the questions you may ask students and the conversations you can have. This does not need to be a script followed directly but acts as a guide to keep the conversations among groups consistent.

To start the conversation, please introduce yourself and your dog to the group and ask the students to introduce themselves to one another. To facilitate conversation, there is a list below of the types of questions you may ask students:

1. Tell me where is home for you? Where are you from?
2. What brought you here to the university?
3. What program are you studying?
4. Tell me about the courses you're taking. Which ones are you enjoying the most?
5. What are things you like to do outside of school? What is it you like about doing that?
6. What do you like about living in our city?
7. What are your favourite places to visit (e.g., parks, restaurants, cafes)?
8. What is something good that has happened this week?
9. What did you do over the weekend?
10. What are your plans for the next week?
11. What are your plans for the summer?
12. What is something you're looking forward to this month?
13. What kind of music do you listen to? Do you have a favourite song? Artist?
14. Have you been to see any shows or concerts recently? If so, what did you go and see? What did you think of the show?
15. What kind of podcasts do you listen to?
16. What books have you read recently? What genre do you like?
17. Have you ever met anyone famous? If so, who? What were they like?
18. Do you have any favourite things you like to cook?
19. Do you have any favourite actors/actresses/artists/comedians?
20. What is a special skill or talent that you have?

(Source: *Anthrozoös*; used with permission)

Two

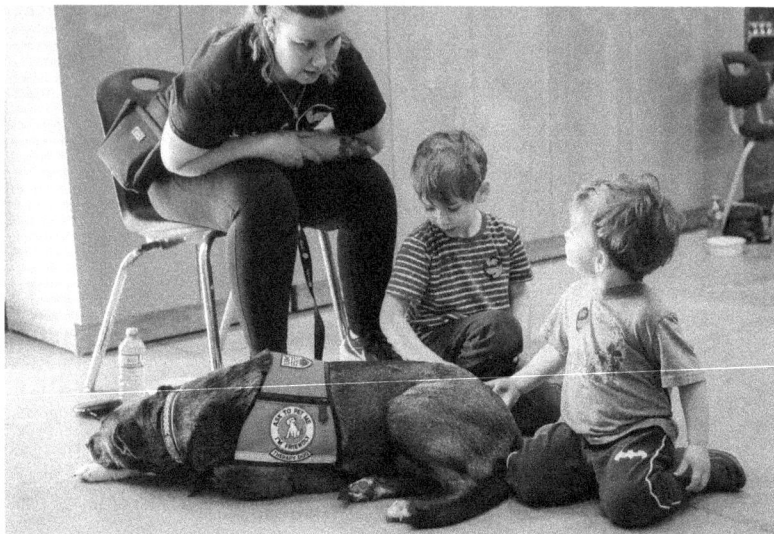

Figure 2.1 Therapy dog-handler Ty interacts with two young children as part of a session as Luna, her therapy dog, relaxes in a lie-down position

Source: Freya L. L. Green Photography; used with permission

Optimizing Therapy Dog-Handler Team Welfare

22

DOI: 10.4324/9781032639284-2

SCENARIO

Therapy Dogs and Humans Helping Each Other and Creating Enjoyment

Billie and their eight-year-old dog named Bentley are an experienced therapy dog-handler team, and they typically visit clients in hospital settings. But Billie is keen to try something new and has heard about after-school library programs that pair up therapy dogs and young readers. Billie knows first-hand how therapy dogs are known as social catalysts bringing people together and has read about their potential to support children's reading. Billie and Bentley enrol in an after-school library program for young readers, and at their first session they are greeted by four young children sitting in a semicircle on a carpeted floor in the centre of the library. Three of the children happily greet Bentley and stroke him gently on the chest before settling in to read their books. Billie notices that the fourth child, a nine-year-old girl named Kira, is at first quiet and reticent to greet Bentley. After some quiet time enjoying the children's attention and stories, Bentley appears playful. Billie is worried that Bentley is becoming too playful and energetic, and some of the children invite Bentley to sit down beside them on the carpet. Instead, Bentley moves around the room and picks up a stuffed toy and drops it near Kira's feet. Kira immediately expresses joy at Bentley's invitation to play! Billie is thrilled to see that Kira and Bentley have made a positive connection and are playing while reading stories; both Bentley and Kira are enjoying the reading session. Billie notes how Bentley and some young readers enjoy quieter interactions with Bentley, whereas Kira enjoys more playful and engaging interactions with Bentley (Figure 2.1). Billie leaves the library rethinking what it means to facilitate a mutually rewarding session between Bentley and young readers – they are dynamic and can involve varied interactions including some unobtrusive movement and play!

QUESTIONS FOR REFLECTION AND DISCUSSION

1. How should after-school library sessions between young readers and a therapy dog be structured? How long should they last? Should they involve brief introductory sessions? Should they include opportunities for both quiet reading and unobtrusive movement and play?

2. What guidance should a handler receive to facilitate mutually rewarding sessions between young readers and a therapy dog? Should a handler be required to receive training before engaging therapy dogs with children in an after-school library program for young readers?

3. What guidance should young readers receive in advance of meeting a therapy dog in an after-school library program? Should a handler be responsible for educating young readers about how to interact with a therapy dog? Should a handler collect information about the children's past experiences with animals?

4. How might we assess if the session is rewarding for both the young reader and the therapy dog? What indicators should a handler consider?

5. To optimize therapy dog welfare and enjoyment, what conditions should be in place for dogs within an after-school library program for young readers?

HISTORY OF CANINE-ASSISTED INTERVENTIONS

As the field of human-animal interactions (HAIs) continues to expand, there is a growing interest in developing opportunities for people to interact with therapy dogs. We provide a historical overview of canine-assisted interventions (CAIs), reviewing early research and outlining a history of organizations spearheading applied programs. We offer an overview of key terminology and outline the salient theories informing our understanding of CAIs. We then discuss the varied components and individuals comprising a CAI and the different research and program designs used to provide opportunities for clients to interact with therapy dog-handler teams. Building on the foundational information shared in Chapter 1, we discuss the findings attesting to the efficacy of CAIs in enhancing well-being outcomes and reducing ill-being outcomes in a variety of clients. We also consider findings reflecting dog-handler teams supporting academic or learning outcomes beyond the well-being context. Our discussion in this chapter serves as a foundation for subsequent discussions of therapy dog-handler team welfare in the chapters that follow.

THE EVER-EXPANDING FIELD OF HAIS

As noted above, HAIs represent a broad umbrella field comprising several interconnected subfields including the human-animal bond (HAB) and animal-assisted interventions (AAIs; e.g., see recent interpretations by Fine & Chastain Griffin, 2022 and Parbery-Clark et al., 2021). The study of HAIs focuses on the reciprocal and interactive relations between humans and animals and considers how humans and animals relate to each other emotionally, psychologically, and physically (Amiot & Bastian, 2015). Often, research in this field is motivated to better understand the learning, health, and psychological benefits of HAIs for both humans and animals. Relatedly, the HAB, a subfield of HAIs, is guided by the hypothesis that "The human-animal bond is a mutually beneficial and dynamic relationship between people and animals that is influenced by behaviours essential to the health and wellbeing of both" (American Veterinary Medical Association 1998, p. 1675). Consistent with this hypothesis, research on the HAB examines the development of social-emotional attachments between people and animals and how the HAB can support the physical, psychological, and social-emotional well-being of both humans and animals (for a review of the health benefits of the HAB for humans, see Fine & Ferrell, 2021).

Further, another subfield of HAI research involves a focus on AAIs. To be clear, there is some overlap between the HAB and AAIs as both operate under the premise that interactions with animals can confer some benefits to human physical and psychological health; however, they are distinct subfields falling under the broader umbrella of HAIs. According to the International Association for Human-Animal Interaction Organizations (IAHAIO, 2018), AAIs involve structured and goal-oriented activities that intentionally include animals in health, education, or human services (e.g., counselling) to promote therapeutic gains in humans (Jegatheesan et al., 2014; Kruger & Serpell, 2006). This definition also includes guidelines for safeguarding the welfare of the animals involved, as published in a white paper by the IAHAIO (2018). Further, AAIs comprise a great deal of variability with respect to their overall structure, specified goals (e.g., therapeutic, educational, emotionally supportive), and the types of animal species involved (e.g., farm animals, dogs, cats, horses, goats, robots that behave like animals; Fine & Ferrell, 2021; Fine et al., 2019; Howell et al., 2022; Parbery-Clark et al., 2021; Santaniello et al., 2020).

CANINE-ASSISTED INTERVENTIONS

Overwhelmingly, AAIs involve therapy dogs who participate in a growing body of research on the impacts of CAIs on human physical and psychological health. CAIs are nested within the broader field of AAIs and continue to see a rise in popularity across contexts and with varied clients. Recently, AAIs that involve therapy dogs and their human handlers are becoming increasingly popular across a multitude of contexts to reduce stress and anxiety, boost mood and provide comfort, facilitate social connections, and support reading and learning (Binfet & Hartwig, 2020). As discussed in Chapter 1, CAIs are typically structured and formalized and can be delivered individually or in group settings (Binfet & Hartwig, 2020). CAIs have been defined as the "bringing together of credentialed canine-assisted intervention teams and members of the public in a specified setting with the purpose of enhancing human well-being" (Binfet & Hartwig, 2020, p. 10).

HISTORY OF HELPING DOGS AND CONTEXTS FOR CAIS

As early as the 19th century, dogs were being trained to facilitate mobility among people who had vision difficulties (Ascarelli, 2010). Early founders of CAIs included Boris Levinson and Elizabeth and Samuel Corson. During the 1960s, Boris Levinson, a child psychologist, unexpectedly observed the positive impact that his dog Jingles had on his young client who was mostly withdrawn and nonverbal. Anecdotally, he noticed that when Jingles was in the room during the therapy sessions, his young client appeared more comfortable and willing to communicate; he witnessed the potential of the HAB to build therapeutic rapport and promote social engagement. Boris Levinson later described Jingles as his co-therapist (Levinson, 1969; 1962), and in 1984, he coined the term *pet therapy*, thus highlighting the value of dogs in a therapeutic context (Levinson, 1987). Further, Elizabeth and Samuel Corson were early (1970s) researchers in the field of CAIs. Empirically, they observed the unexpected and positive impact of dogs on clients with psychiatric disorders including one patient who was quiet and selectively mute (Corson et al., 1977). They noticed that when the dogs were included as part of the daily programming the psychiatric clients appeared more communicative with each other and staff. Notably, the Corsons coined the term *social lubricant*

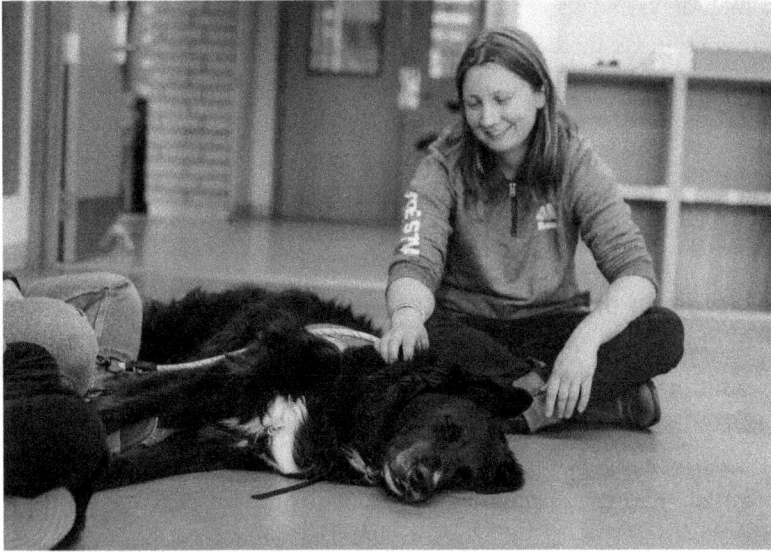

Figure 2.2 Therapy dog Forrest, a Border Collie mix, feels safe and secure enough to fall asleep while receiving physical attention from Annie, a graduate student

Source: F. L. L. Green Photography; used with permission

describing the presence of the dogs as helping to foster feelings of warmth and friendliness and forge social connections among clients and staff (Figure 2.2).

Today, CAIs have evolved since the work of the early founders from involving mainly one therapist and one dog, as was the case with Boris Levinson and his companion dog Jingles, to including varied applications. Indeed, as highlighted above and in Chapter 1, today's CAIs generally include dogs working with varied clients, guided by different goals, and across a multitude of contexts. Here, we acknowledge many categories of working dogs including therapy dogs, visitation dogs, service dogs, emotional support dogs, and companion dogs (for a comprehensive discussion of key terms used for animals working in supportive roles, see Howell et al., 2022). Given this book's focus on therapy dog-handler teams, we rely heavily on our familiarity and experience with therapy dogs and draw on research with this category of working dog to support our insights and practice recommendations. Today, therapy dog-handler teams have evolved to include varied applications which can involve one or many clients across contexts including but not limited to airports, university and college campuses, elementary schools, crisis centres, counselling, medical and dental offices, hospitals, public libraries, funeral homes, long-term care facilities, homeless shelters, recovery centres, and military bases (for a comprehensive discussion of the varied applications of therapy dog-handler teams, see Binfet & Hartwig, 2020).

HISTORY OF ORGANIZATIONS SPEARHEADING DEVELOPMENTS IN CAIS

In addition to the work of early founders such as Boris Levinson and Elizabeth and Samuel Corson, several organizations were pivotal in spearheading developments in the field of CAIs (see Figure 2.3) and their efforts are ongoing and remain impactful. Some of these organizations aim to unite researchers, professionals, policymakers, and members of the public who are interested in HAIs to promote dialogue, education, and best practices in AAIs and disseminate research findings. Still, other organizations are more practice-oriented aiming to train and certify successful therapy dog-handler teams. Significantly, all these organizations share a common mission to promote positive interactions between humans and animals, raise awareness about the benefits of animals to human health, support high-quality research and best practices in HAIs and AAIs including CAIs, and improve and

Key Developments Over Time

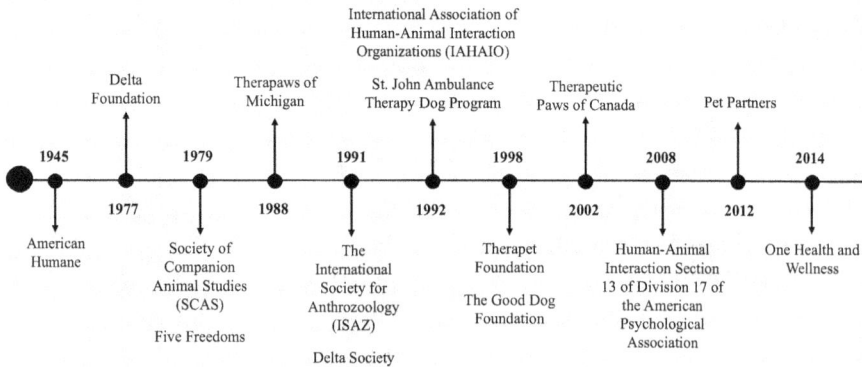

Figure 2.3 Timeline of key developments from 1945 to 2014 in CAIs

advocate for the welfare of animals (see Figure 2.3 for a timeline of key developments in CAIs).

American Humane

As early as 1877, American Humane was established, and in 1945, a therapy dog program was developed for recovering the Second World War veterans. Today, American Humane is committed to protecting and promoting the welfare of animals, including therapy dogs. Importantly, the organization supports animal-assisted therapy programs led by trained and certified handlers who require animals to undergo regular health and behavioural assessments, and who comply with the Code of Ethics for animal-assisted activities and therapy (Mission, n.d.-a).

Delta Foundation/Delta Society/Pet Partners

In 1977, a team of veterinarians and medical practitioners established the Delta Foundation, with Dr. Michael McCullough as their first president. This team included Dr. Bill McCullough, Dr. Leo K. Bustad, Dr. R. K. Anderson, Dr. Stanley L. Diesch, and Dr. Joe Quigley, and their goal in establishing the Delta Foundation was to study the HAB with a focus on "The Delta Triangle": the animal, the client, and the veterinarian. In 1981, The Delta Foundation was reconfigured and established as the Delta Society, with Dr. Bill McCullough as the first founding president. The Delta Society was pivotal in promoting the HAB by creating the American Veterinary Medical Association HAB Task Force and establishing Anthrozoös, a peer-reviewed research journal which has since become a well-respected publisher of high-quality HAI research. In 1991, the Pet Partners program was established as part of the Delta Society's mission to advance community awareness about the HAB. Pet Partners was established as the first standardized training in animal-assisted activities and therapy for healthcare workers and volunteers. Today, Pet Partners' mandate is to certify and register therapy animal teams which are comprised of a trained handler and their animal (many of which are dogs). These therapy animal-handler teams are then well equipped to make visits and engage in various activities to provide comfort and support to people in varied contexts (e.g., schools, long-term care facilities, and hospitals). Additionally, Pet Partners engages in research and education to advance the understanding of the benefits of the

HAB. In 2012, the *Delta Society* officially changed its name to *Pet Partners* to better align with its mission of promoting and supporting research and education on the benefits (e.g., educational, therapeutic) of the HAB (*About*, n.d.). For a comprehensive discussion of the defining moments and significant individuals responsible for the evolution of *Pet Partners* from the *Delta Foundation* and *Delta Society*, see Fine et al. (2023).

The International Society for Anthrozoology

The first meeting of the International Society for Anthrozoology (ISAZ) was held in 1991, with Dr. Erika Friedmann elected as the first president of the society. The mission of ISAZ is to support and develop the growing community of researchers and scholars working in the field of Anthrozoology (the study of HAIs) by promoting international research collaborations. Towards this goal, ISAZ continues to host annual conferences with conference locations being held in countries around the world. Further, in 2002, *Anthrozoös* (a multidisciplinary journal of the interactions of people and animals) became the official journal of ISAZ, and since this time, the society has continued to publish high-quality research on people's interactions with animals and the impact on both human and animal welfare (*Mission*, n.d.-b).

Human-Animal Interaction Section 13 of Division 17 of the American Psychological Association

In 2008, the Human-Animal Interaction Section 13 of Division 17 (Society of Counseling Psychology) was established by the American Psychological Association (APA; Beck et al., 2018). The Section on Human-Animal Interaction: Research & Practice is committed to promoting and supporting scholarly and professional activities that advance our understanding of HAIs as they are connected to the discipline of psychology. The Human-Animal Interaction Section 13 of Division 17 organized the development of the *Human-Animal Interaction Bulletin* (an online, open-access publication now titled *Human-Animal Interactions*) and is associated (since 2016) with a special section devoted to HAI research in the *Journal of Applied Developmental Science*.

Society of Companion Animal Studies

In 1979, the *Society of Companion Animal Studies* (SCAS) was established to promote the continual improvement of both human and animal well-being by facilitating and supporting HAIs. The society adopts a *One Health One Welfare* worldview that advocates for the interconnectedness of animal welfare, human well-being, and our shared environment. Towards this goal, the SCAS aims to encourage and support best practices in AAIs, to support the HAB, and to make available training and resources for facilitating mutually rewarding HAIs. The society compiles and disseminates research-informed findings about the health benefits of HAIs for members, healthcare practitioners, animal welfare experts, and other practitioners working with animals (*About us*, n.d.-b).

International Association of Human-Animal Interaction Organizations

Established in 1992, the IAHAIO offers an international and collaborative platform for researchers, professionals, policymakers, members of the public, and other organizations to advance research, education, and practice in the field of HAIs (*Mission and goals*, n.d.). Towards this goal, IAHAIO regularly hosts international conferences, meets yearly, and publishes research articles in an open-access journal and, importantly, addresses critical issues in the field including best practices in AAIs.

Therapaws of Michigan

Established in 1988, *Therapaws* aims to promote and foster the HAB through canine-assisted therapy in both educational and therapeutic contexts (*About us*, n.d.-c). *Therapaws's* mission is to advance the therapeutic benefits of the HAB, and towards this goal, they place certified therapy dog-handler teams (through Alliance of Therapy Dogs) with people in varied community contexts including hospitals, healthcare facilities, schools, and public libraries, with the goal of promoting mutually beneficial interactions between people and dogs.

St. John Ambulance Therapy Dog Program

Established in 1992, *St. John Ambulance Therapy Dog Program* works with teams of volunteers and their dogs and offers visits to people in varied community settings (e.g., hospitals, seniors' and nursing residences, schools, public libraries). The program's mission is to provide people who are lonely or ill or who reside in long-term care or mental health facilities with comfort and companionship by interacting with trained therapy dogs. The overarching goal of these interactions between people and trained therapy dogs is to enhance the quality of human health and well-being (*Therapy dog program*, n.d.).

Therapet Foundation

The *Therapet Foundation* was established in 1998 and is broadly committed to raising awareness of the benefits of AAT among healthcare professionals, educators, and communities. Like the *St. John Ambulance Therapy Dog Program*, *Therapet Foundation* works with teams of highly trained and certified teams of volunteers and their companion animals (mostly dogs) to support and comfort people within the community. The organization also offers educational expertise and training and certification programs for the successful administration of AAT and animal-assisted activities (*About therapet*, n.d.).

The Good Dog Foundation

The *Good Dog Foundation* was established in 1998 with the goal of advancing the field of AAIs. Their mandate is to prepare dog-human teams so that they can support and comfort people in need of assistance. The foundation comprises experts in diverse fields including psychology, veterinary medicine, and AAI, and trains and certifies volunteers and professionals to work with their dogs to provide support in diverse settings, including hospitals, schools, nursing homes, and other facilities (*About us*, n.d.-a). The foundation is also involved in collaborative research with hospitals and universities to promote mutually rewarding therapy dog-handler team interactions and successful applications to community initiatives.

Therapeutic Paws of Canada

Therapeutic Paws of Canada was established in 2002 and is committed to enhancing the quality of human life, health, and well-being by offering visits with volunteer handlers and their qualified companion animals, which consist mostly of dogs and cats (*Our story*, n.d.). These therapy animal-handler visits are designed to offer therapeutic benefits to vulnerable people in varied contexts who need emotional support and companionship (e.g., seniors, children, and youth).

ANIMAL WELFARE AND CURRENT TRENDS IN CAIS: SCHOLARLY PUBLICATIONS

Here, we note several other key developments that foregrounded an increasing focus on animal welfare concerns in HAIs, AAIs, and CAIs. Notably, in 1979, the Five Freedoms of animal welfare were developed with the original goal of safeguarding animal welfare in livestock (UK Farm Animal Welfare Council). Globally, many professionals (e.g., veterinarians) and organizations (e.g., Royal Society for the Prevention of Cruelty to Animals) have applied the Five Freedoms as a standard when considering the welfare of domestic and therapy animals. The Five Freedoms include (1) freedom from hunger, thirst, and malnutrition; (2) freedom from discomfort; (3) freedom from pain, injury, or disease; (4) freedom from fear and distress; and (5) freedom to express normal behaviour. Recently, scholars and researchers have extended the Five Freedoms model beyond providing benchmark standards of care to also include positive affective states in animals and animals' potential to flourish (Barker & Gee, 2021; McBride & Baugh, 2022; Ng et al., 2015).

Yet another notable development followed in 2014 when the IAHAIO published a white paper including not only definitions for animal-assisted activities but considerations and guidelines for safeguarding the well-being of animals working in these contexts (IAHAIO, 2018; Jegatheesan et al., 2014). Still, more recently, many researchers, professionals (e.g., veterinarians, mental health workers), and organizations have adopted a One Health and Wellness approach which recognizes the interconnections between human welfare, animal welfare, and the integrity of the environment (Chalmers & Dell, 2015; Peralta & Fine, 2021; Pinillos, 2018). In this way, a One Health and Wellness approach calls for professional practice that promotes both human and animal welfare and emphasizes environmental stewardship as fundamental to this goal.

Owing to the ongoing efforts of various organizations and dedicated researchers, practitioners, and advocates, the field of CAIs has come a long way and has seen many key developments. See Appendix 2.1 for an illustration of key animal therapy organizations (the majority of which include dogs) around the world. Significantly, there is growing awareness about animals' complex lived experiences and mounting concern for ethical practice and animal welfare among researchers, practitioners, and community members alike. As a testament to these concerns, and as discussed in Chapter 1, we are witnessing significant changes in how AAIs and CAIs are implemented with a trend towards greater attention to defining protocols for safeguarding animal well-being in interactions with humans (for a review, see Fine et al., 2019). Further, research articles devoted specifically to the study of animal welfare and ethical practice in AAIs and CAIs continue to grow in numbers. Notably, the field of AAIs and CAIs is seeing the publication of new papers with a focus on animal (canine) welfare, and we now have the first book ever focusing on the animal's perspective and welfare in the context of AAIs and CAIs (Peralta & Fine, 2021). Also, as illustrated in Chapter 1, there is a growing trend for published research to include information about animal (i.e., therapy dog) participants, often describing them in as much detail as the human participants. It is also more common practice for researchers to report the details of animal welfare concerns as part of their published papers. The issue of animal ethics in research protocols will be addressed further in Chapter 3.

In this regard, there is growing recognition that best practices in CAIs (and HAIs and AAIs, more generally) will need to include a focus on animal welfare and ethical practice. Trevathan-Minnis et al. (2023) qualitatively surveyed 186 respondents from across 17 groups who were involved in HAIs from varied groups including health and mental healthcare providers, animal trainers and behaviourists, and people working in higher education. Results suggested that animal welfare concerns ranked high as an area of critical need for future research and practice in the field of HAIs. In another study (Ameli & Krämer, 2023), professionals who were working directly in the field of AAIs assigned a high priority to animal welfare concerns and rated themselves as being able to reliably identify animal welfare-related signs in their AAI practice and to follow up by taking appropriate actions to safeguard and optimize animal welfare. In their review of AAIs, Fine and colleagues (2019) argue that significant advances in the field of AAIs will be realized when therapy animal *and* human welfare are prioritized at all stages of the intervention (i.e., before, during, and after). We agree with Fine and his colleagues on this latter point and position therapy dog-handler teams as cohesive and dynamic; this definition will be further expanded in Chapter 3. Importantly, we argue that the welfare of both partners of the therapy dog-handler team is mutually constitutive and critical to the success of CAIs. At this point, we acknowledge the growing body of research on the welfare concerns of diverse animals (e.g., farm, cats, goats, etc.) in AAIs (Sirovica & von Keyserlingk, 2023; von Keyserlingk & Weary, 2017); however, in this book, we focus our discussion on therapy dog-handler welfare and best practices in the context of CAIs. The above-noted welfare-related developments in AAI and CAI research and practice will be considered in greater detail in the chapters that follow.

THEORIES UNDERGIRDING CAIS

We draw on several theories outlining potential mechanisms to help us understand the observed benefits of CAIs for both humans and canines. These theories range from mainly cross-disciplinary to inherently interdisciplinary in focus and are informed by advances in social, developmental, and evolutionary psychology, biology, critical animal studies, and animal studies or posthumanism. Our book's focus is inherently interdisciplinary, and we draw mostly on the *biophilia hypothesis* (Kellert & Wilson, 1993; Wilson, 1984); *biopsychosocial theory and attachment theory* (e.g., Gee et al., 2021); *social support theory* (Cobb, 1976; Cohen & Wills, 1985; Schaefer et al., 1981); research on *motivation, engagement, and learning* (Gee et al., 2017; Wohlfarth et al., 2013); and interdisciplinary frameworks such as *animal studies or posthumanism* (Haraway, 2008) and *critical animal studies* (Matsuoka & Sorenson, 2018).

Biophilia Hypothesis

To help us understand the appeal of CAIs and the associated benefits for human health and well-being, we draw conceptually on the biophilia hypothesis. The biophilia hypothesis asserts that people have an "innate tendency to focus on life and lifelike processes" (Wilson, 1984, p. 1) and that people strive to connect with nature including animals. Serpell (1996) notes that animals offer a live stimulus which serves to draw a person's interest and focus his or her attention and, in this way, contributes to an overall calming effect. Researchers have suggested that interacting with calm animals is engaging and can promote feelings of security and calm in humans (Julius et al., 2013).

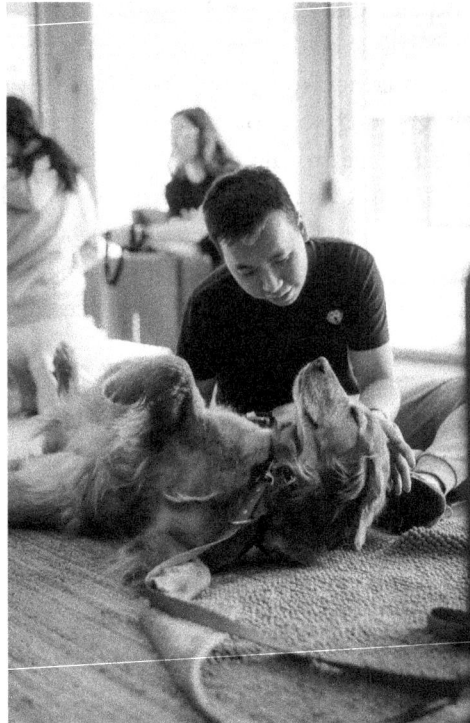

Figure 2.4 Therapy dog Hana, a Golden Retriever, lies on her back and enjoys receiving physical attention from Hugo, a university student; both the therapy dog and the student are content and gazing at each other
Source: F. L. L. Green Photography; used with permission

This might explain the mechanisms through which engaging with a therapy dog reduces stress and anxiety and promotes positive affective states. Further, in the context of CAIs, we must consider the concept of emotional contagion between the therapy dog and handler – that dogs can "feel and catch" their handlers' emotions (and vice versa) (Katayama et al., 2019). We argue that the success of CAIs for humans is predicated on the capacity for both agents comprising the therapy dog-handler team to dynamically share and project feelings of calm, contentment, and a general sense of well-being (Figure 2.4).

Biopsychosocial and Attachment Theories

We also draw on *biopsychosocial* (Gee et al., 2021) and *attachment* (Bowlby, 1969) theories to help us understand the appeal of CAIs and the associated benefits for human health and well-being. According to biological theories, humans' relationships with domestic animals are rooted in evolutionary, psychological, and physiological processes (Beck, 2014). As evidence of humans' biological preparedness to connect with animals, Beck and Katcher (1996) point to humans' attraction to neotenous features in young animals which include juvenile features such as large eyes, rounded forehead, and ears, and shortened muzzle. Further, attachment theory also highlights the need for humans and animals to protect and to be protected – they are biologically predisposed to protect their offspring to ensure their survival (Bowlby, 1969; Sable, 1995). An attachment figure can offer a secure base from which young children and animals can safely explore their diverse environments. There is a corresponding biological predisposition for young children and animals to seek and maintain physical proximity to a sensitive and responsive attachment figure who can offer protection and care – this is an adaptive response particularly when the environment is less predictable (Figure 2.5).

Researchers have shown that direct, social touching and intimate contact between humans and animals can promote the development of the HAB (for a discussion, see Fine & Ferrell, 2021). As noted previously, animals can also help to create a calm and comforting ambience for their human companions. A *biopsychosocial* approach submits that people's intimate interactions with dogs (and animals) may have important impacts on people's physical and psychological health and well-being (Gee et al., 2021). Notably, Gee and colleagues (2021) suggest biological mechanisms can help to explain recent findings supporting the stress-buffering benefits for people interacting with animals (Barker et al., 2016; Handlin et al., 2011; Janssens et al., 2021). They suggest that interacting with dogs can reduce stress and increase positive affective states by reducing cortisol levels (a hormone associated with stress) and releasing oxytocin (a hormone associated with attachment and affiliation – the *love* or *bonding* hormone; Rault et al., 2017). Mutual eye gazing between dogs and their human companions has also been linked to increases in oxytocin levels in both dogs and humans, supporting a positive oxytocin loop (Nagasawa et al., 2015; Odendaal & Mientjes, 2003). As argued by Gee et al. (2021), these biological effects may contribute positively to human physical and psychological health.

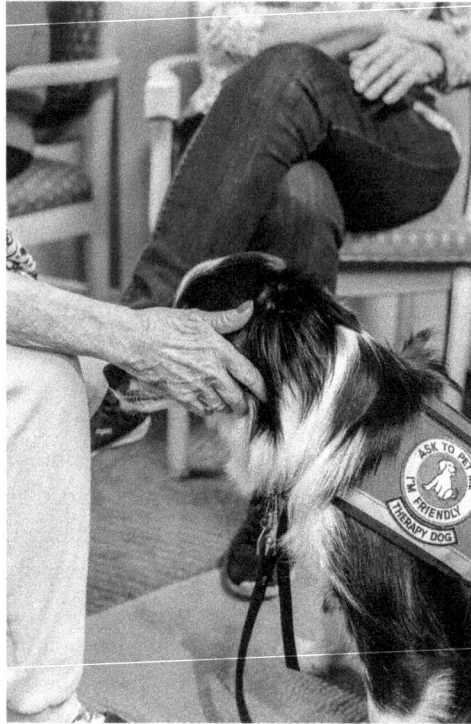

Figure 2.5 Border Collie Pie, a therapy dog, rests her head in the hands of a senior lady

Source: F. L. L. Green Photography; used with permission

In the context of CAIs, we must consider recent research suggesting that humans and companion dogs can share and exhibit strong attachments towards one another (e.g., Payne et al., 2015; Thielke & Udell, 2020). According to Fine (2014), the development of the HAB relies heavily on the strength of an animal's attachment to humans, much like the attachment relationships shared between infants and their caregivers. Here, we highlight the importance of considering the strength of the attachment relationship between therapy dogs and their handlers. Significantly, we note that therapy dog-handler teams might vary widely in the type and strength of their shared attachment. Here again, we argue that the success of CAIs for human health and welfare rests on the premise that both agents comprising the therapy dog-handler team share a strong and positive attachment relationship.

Social Support Theory

Another way to understand the appeal of CAIs and the associated benefits for human health and well-being is to consider the positive impacts of social support. *Social support theory* suggests that social relationships provide a buffer against anxiety, depression, and other related illnesses (Cobb, 1976). Having a supportive network of friends, family, and peers can foster positive health effects (Cobb 1976; Hupcey 1998) and can mediate between stress and physical and psychological health (Schaefer et al., 1981; Wilks & Spivey, 2010). This model of social support has been applied to explain the physiological and psychological benefits of interacting with companion animals (Fine & Weaver 2018; O'Haire 2010). Studies show that when people are accompanied by a companion animal, they are perceived by others as less threatening, and more relaxed, happier, friendlier, and more desirable as acquaintances or friends (Eddy et al., 2001). In this way, animals can serve as "social lubricants" or catalysts to facilitate communication and rapport between people and may ease discomfort in an anxiety-inducing context and support positive health and well-being (Guest et al., 2006; Kruger & Serpell, 2010). Within the context of CAIs, therapy dog-handler teams act as "social lubricants" or catalysts to facilitate communication and rapport between people (Guest et al., 2006; Kruger & Serpell, 2010). In this way, therapy dog-handler teams may ease discomfort in an anxiety-inducing context and support positive health and well-being. Still, the success of CAIs will be optimized when both parties – therapy dog and handler – share and project a supportive relationship.

Research on Motivation, Engagement, and Learning, and CAIs

We also draw conceptually on research related to motivation, engagement, and learning (Gee et al., 2017; Wohlfarth et al., 2013) to help us understand the appeal of CAIs and the associated benefits for human learning and well-being. Gee and colleagues (2017) propose a unified framework in which the effect of AAIs (and CAIs) on people's learning and social-emotional well-being is mediated by motivation and self-efficacy, engagement/attention and executive functions, self-regulation and stress coping, and social interactions. In the context of CAIs, therapy dogs might have an indirect effect on learning by increasing people's motivation and self-efficacy and enhancing engagement/attention and executive functions. In this way, therapy dogs might help to increase students' implicit motives by arousing their capacities to orient, select, and energize activities such as reading to a therapy dog (Wohlfarth et al., 2013). Further, integrating a calm and supportive therapy dog-handler as part of a CAI can help to reduce learners' stress and sensory overstimulation and activate their cognitive energy (Schuck & Fine, 2017); this might be especially important for learners who have attention-deficit hyperactivity disorder or other learning difficulties. We reiterate here that the success of CAIs for human learning and well-being rests largely on the capacity for both the therapy dog and their handler to dynamically share and project feelings of calm, contentment, and a general sense of well-being.

Interdisciplinary Frameworks: Animal Studies or Posthumanism and Critical Animal Studies

Lastly, we also draw conceptually on interdisciplinary frameworks such as animal studies or posthumanism (Haraway, 2008) and critical animal studies (Matsuoka & Sorenson, 2018). These frameworks outline innovative perspectives on animals and HAIs (for a discussion, see Adams, 2018) and directly challenge speciesism and anthropocentrism. In this way, these frameworks challenge traditional boundaries between humans and animals (Haraway, 2008; Shapiro, 2020), and embrace a *relational ontology* wherein the relations between humans and animals are conceptualized as mutually constitutive (Haraway, 2008; Shapiro, 2020). These ideas correspond with recent calls in the field of HAI for a repositioning of animals (and therapy dogs) that highlights reciprocity in animals' interactions with humans and is consistent with an ever-increasing focus on animal agency and welfare in the context of AAIs and CAIs (Ng et al., 2015). In the context of CAIs, therapy dogs and handlers alike are considered key agents working as a "cohesive team" and whose positive contribution to human health and well-being is optimized when both animal and human welfare is prioritized. We consider some of these exciting ideas in Chapter 8 when we discuss current trends and future directions in optimizing therapy dog-handler teams in the context of CAIs.

Recall in the scenario at the outset of this chapter that Billie, a handler, is curious about the promise of therapy dogs to support young readers in an after-school library setting. Billie is curious about the efficacy and benefits of CAIs to support reading enjoyment and motivation, and they is keen to facilitate a mutually rewarding and playful session between their dog Bentley and Kira, a young reader who is initially quiet and reticent to greet Bentley. We now consider emerging findings on the benefits of CAIs for human well-being and the implications for therapy dog well-being (Figure 2.6).

To begin, throughout this chapter, we have alluded to the varied components and agents comprising a CAI (e.g., client and therapy dog-handler team) and of the different research and program designs

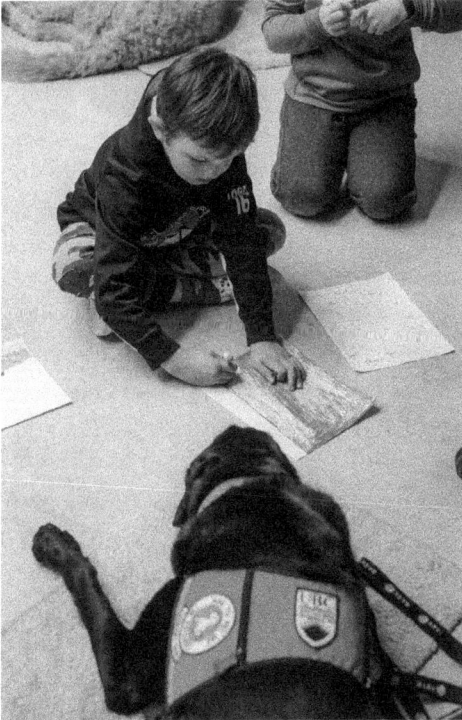

Figure 2.6 Therapy dog Lexi, a black Labrador wearing a red vest, rests comfortably and watches as two nearby children engage in a drawing activity

Source: F. L. L. Green Photography; used with permission

used to provide opportunities for clients to interact with therapy dog-handler teams. Contributors include researchers or professionals organizing and delivering a CAI for a specified goal, the client(s), and therapy dog-handler team; in our scenario at the outset of this chapter, the setting involves an after-school library and the individuals to consider include Billie (handler), Bentley (therapy dog), and several young readers (including Kira); in this context, Bentley and Billie join to form a cohesive and dynamic therapy dog-handler team. Here we reiterate that CAIs comprise a great deal of variability with respect to their overall structure (i.e., one-time visit or several weekly visits), specified goals (e.g., therapeutic, educational, and emotionally supportive), types of activities (e.g., reading to a dog, training a shelter dog as part of a prison program, and physical rehabilitation), and type of clients involved (e.g., young or senior clients, military veterans with posttraumatic stress disorder, children who have disabilities, and other vulnerable clients). CAIs also vary in terms of the number of clients involved, as they can be delivered one-on-one, with several clients, or with a group of people as part of community building exercises or for people who are experiencing a traumatic event *en masse* such as following a natural disaster event (Fine & Ferrell, 2021; Fine et al., 2019; Howell et al., 2022; Parbery-Clark et al., 2021; Santaniello et al., 2020). Finally, the settings of CAIs are also varied and as noted previously can include therapy dog-handler teams visiting hospitals and dental offices, long-term and mental healthcare facilities, prison facilities, public libraries, and other recreational and workplace contexts (for a comprehensive discussion of the varied contexts of CAIs, see Binfet & Hartwig, 2020).

Recently, we have seen an explosion in studies examining the impact of HAIs for human learning and physical and psychological health (for a review, see Gee & Mueller, 2019). Regarding AAIs and activities, a growing number of studies demonstrate the academic, social, and emotional benefits for humans across the lifespan (for reviews, see Hall et al., 2016; Nimer & Lundahl, 2007; Reilly et al., 2020; Sandt, 2020). Studies are more rigorous than ever as researchers continue to refine their designs and employ innovative methodologies to more accurately assess the benefits and drawbacks associated with HAIs and AAIs for human and animal health and well-being. Here, too, the field of CAIs has come a long way as anecdotal evidence has been largely replaced by rigorous scientific findings. In the section that follows, we briefly summarize some of the documented benefits arising from CAIs for humans (for a comprehensive discussion of the benefits of CAIs for human physical and psychological health, see Binfet & Hartwig, 2020), and we also consider the implications for canine welfare.

Physical and Well-Being Benefits: Self-Reports

Using self-reports, studies have also documented numerous benefits of CAIs for human learning, and social and emotional well-being across the lifespan (for a review, see Gee et al., 2021). Initial evidence suggests positive outcomes for university or college students when they interact with therapy dogs including reduced homesickness and increased campus connectedness (Binfet & Passmore, 2016), reductions in perceived stress and improvements in school belonging (Banks et al., 2018; Barker et al., 2016; Binfet, 2017; Ward-Griffin et al., 2018), and positive changes in mood (Crossman et al., 2015; Grajfoner et al., 2017; Pendry et al., 2018). In one study, students who interacted with therapy dogs for eight weeks reported significantly less homesickness and greater satisfaction with life as compared to the students in the wait-listed control group (Binfet et al., 2018). Further, the positive impacts of CAIs might translate to benefits in learning and emotional well-being among university students. For instance, in a randomized controlled trial by Pendry and colleagues (2018), students assigned to the combined standard stress manage ment program and dog interaction condition reported significantly higher levels of enjoyment, usefulness, self-regulation, and behaviour change than students assigned to either one of these conditions alone. It is worth noting that research indicates that even brief and infrequent interactions with therapy dogs may decrease perceived stress and increase perceived happiness among college students (Ward-Griffin et al., 2018; Wood et al., 2017).

Researchers have also found that brief, unstructured interactions with a therapy dog can significantly reduce self-reported anxiety and distress levels among patients receiving emergency care (Kline et al., 2019), plus reduce self-reported anxiety and negative mood and increase self-reported positive mood among post-secondary students (Crossman et al., 2015). In one study, undergraduate students who had experienced trauma reported decreases in depressive symptoms when receiving psychotherapy in the presence of a therapy dog (Hunt & Chizkov, 2014). In another study of children aged 10–13 years findings showed that brief, unstructured interactions with dogs boosted children's positive emotions and reduced anxiety (Crossman et al., 2020). Further, there is some evidence that CAIs can help to reduce depression and increase quality of life in older adults with mild to moderate dementia (Travers et al., 2013) and reduce anxiety in adults with Alzheimer's (Mossello et al., 2011), as assessed by medical and/or mental health professionals.

Additionally, researchers have underscored the benefits of engaging with companion dogs for neurodiverse children such as reducing anxiety (Wright et al., 2015) and improving mood, sleep, and problematic behaviour among children who have autism spectrum disorder (Burrows et al., 2008; Carlisle, 2014) – as reported by the children's caregivers. Schuck and colleagues (2015) found that, according to parental reports, children with attention-deficit hyperactivity disorder who received cognitive behavioural therapy with a CAI showed greater reductions in the severity of their symptoms as compared to children who received cognitive behavioural therapy without the CAI. Last, initial evidence suggests that engaging with a therapy dog has a number of cognitive and academic benefits for young learners including improved reading performance (Hall et al., 2016), improved speed and accuracy on cognitive and motor skills tasks when compared to interacting with a stuffed dog or human (Gee et al., 2015), and greater frontal lobe activity in the presence of a real dog, versus a robotic dog, thus indicating a higher level of neuropsychological attention (Hediger & Turner, 2014).

The evidence clearly indicates the self-perceived benefits of engaging with therapy dogs in CAIs for human health and well-being. However, little is known about how these engagements are experienced by the dogs involved in CAIs. We ask, "How do therapy dogs experience CAIs? Do therapy dogs enjoy their structured interactions with humans? Does the structure of CAIs (i.e., length and duration) place increased demands on therapy dogs, possibly compromising their well-being in CAIs?" While some research suggests that longer, structured interactions with therapy dogs are ideal for enhancing human health and well-being, some questions remain: "Are brief or longer CAI sessions better for therapy dogs?" "What are best practices in CAIs to optimize therapy dog welfare and flourishing?" We must consider that a successful CAI will vary for each person and will be experienced differently by each therapy dog. For example, recall that in the scenario at the outset of this chapter, Kira (the young reader) is described as quiet and reticent to greet Bentley (the therapy dog), which is until Bentley drops a stuffed toy at Kira's feet and invites her to play. Through play, both Kira and Bentley make a positive and mutually rewarding connection with Kira reading stories to Bentley; they are both enjoying the reading session. Here, we recognize that successful CAIs can take different shapes and forms, with some being calming and others being more interactive and playful in nature. As we will discuss further in Chapter 5, we must also consider how therapy dogs experience CAIs: *Do they enjoy participating in CAIs?* and *Do they experience them as rewarding?* (Winkle & Johnson Binder, 2024).

Physical Health Benefits: Biomarker Indicators

Recent studies have documented the positive physical health benefits associated with CAIs. Studies have shown reductions in markers of stress during the presence of a dog among young children undergoing a physical examination (Nagengast et al., 1997), decreased systolic blood pressure in hospitalized children (Tsai et al., 2010), reductions in pain in children in a pediatric setting (Braun et al., 2009) and among chronic pain adult patients (Marcus et al., 2013), and lowered salivary biomarkers for stress among children who are engaged in forensic interviews related to sexual abuse allegations (Krause-Parello & Friedmann, 2014). Still, other studies have shown reductions in salivary cortisol among university students attending an animal visitation program (Pendry & Vandagriff, 2019), and among neurodiverse children, with children who have autism spectrum disorder showing reductions in cortisol awakening response following the introduction of a service dog to their family (Viau et al., 2010).

According to the *biopsychosocial theory* (Gee et al., 2021), these biological benefits are likely owing to the physical contact and touch that therapy dogs afford people. Indeed, initial evidence underscores the importance of touch in the context of CAIs. In a randomized controlled trial (Binfet et al., 2021), only undergraduate students in the touch versus no-touch dog condition reported significant improvements on all measures of well-being (e.g., flourishing, happiness, loneliness, stress, social connectedness, positive and negative affect). In another randomized controlled trial, salivary cortisol levels were lowest among undergraduate students in the hands-on petting of dogs and cats, versus the observation of others petting dogs and cats, the viewing images of dogs and cats, or the wait-list conditions (Pendry & Vandagriff, 2019). Further, Beetz and colleagues (2011) explored the role of touch in a sample of young boys aged 7–12 years and found that increased physical touching of a real dog (versus a toy dog or interaction with a friendly human) was associated with lowered salivary cortisol levels. In contrast to these latter findings, Mueller and colleagues (2021) explored the role of touch in adolescents with anxiety and did not find evidence that interacting with a real dog – with or without opportunities for physical touch – was associated with reductions in anxiety or autonomic reactivity.

Clearly, there is emerging evidence suggesting that touch might enhance people's well-being in the context of CAIs. However, little is known about how physical contact and touch are received by therapy dogs in CAIs. We ask, "How do therapy dogs experience human touch in CAIs? Does touch from an unfamiliar human versus a familiar handler change the experience in any way for therapy dogs? Does human touch place increased demands on therapy dogs, possibly compromising their enjoyment of CAIs?" While some research suggests that physical contact and touch are good for humans, we must ask, "Is touch always good for the therapy dog?" and "Is touch good for all therapy dogs?" We must consider that the quality of human touch varies for each person and will be experienced differently by each therapy dog. Returning to the scenario at the outset of this chapter in which Kira (the young reader) is described as quiet and reticent to greet Bentley (the therapy dog), we must also consider how Bentley experienced this type of quiet interaction. Perhaps Bentley enjoyed Kira's quiet, gradual greeting characterized by ambient co-presence? Once again, we consider whether Bentley's welfare was optimized and if he experienced the session as rewarding. We also point to the importance of attending to diversity among young people (e.g., children who have attention-deficit hyperactivity disorder, externalizing behavioural problems such as conduct disorder, or previous experiences of animal cruelty) and the implications for optimizing therapy dog-handler welfare in the context of CAIs.

CONCLUSION

The field of CAIs has come a long way owing to the ongoing efforts of various organizations and dedicated researchers, practitioners, and advocates. Rapid and significant developments have occurred in the field of CAI research and practice, with new insights into ethical practice and ways to safeguard and optimize canine welfare. In this chapter, we offered a historical overview of CAIs, reviewing early research and outlining a history of organizations spearheading applied programs. We then reviewed key terminology and considered various theories and potential mechanisms to inform our understanding of CAIs. Additionally, we considered the varied components and individuals comprising a CAI and the different research and program designs used to provide opportunities for clients to interact with therapy dog-handler teams. Lastly, we discussed the findings attesting to the efficacy of CAIs in enhancing well-being outcomes and reducing ill-being outcomes in a variety of clients. In Chapter 3, we delve deeper into the consideration of canine welfare, define the concept of therapy dog-handler team "welfare," and explore the concept of emotional contagion between handlers and dogs. We hope that researchers, educators, and practitioners alike will consider how they might facilitate mutually rewarding CAIs in which clients and therapy dog-handler teams can flourish.

REFERENCES

About. (n.d.). Pet Partners. Retrieved June 12, 2024, from https://petpartners.org/about/

About therapet. (n.d.). TheraPet | Animal Assisted Therapy. Retrieved June 12, 2024, from https://therapet.org/about/our-vision-values/

About us. (n.d.-a). The Good Dog Foundation. Retrieved June 12, 2024, from https://thegooddogfoundation.org/about-us/#mission

About us. (n.d.-b). Society for Companion Animal Studies. Retrieved June 12, 2024, from https://www.scas.org.uk/about/

About us. (n.d.-c). Therapaws of Michigan, Inc. Retrieved June 12, 2024, from https://therapaws.org/about-us/

Adams, M. (2018). Towards a critical psychology of human–animal relations. *Social and Personality Psychology Compass*, 12(4), 1–14. https://doi.org/10.1111/spc3.12375

Ameli, K., Braun, T. F., & Krämer, S. (2023). Animal-assisted interventions and animal welfare—an exploratory survey in Germany. *Animals*, 13(8), 1324. https://doi.org/10.3390/ani13081324

American Veterinary Medical Association. (1998). Statement from the committee on the human-animal bond. *Journal of the American Veterinary Medical Association*, 212(11), 1675.

Amiot, C. E., & Bastian, B. (2015). Toward a psychology of human-animal relations. *Psychological Bulletin*, 141(1), 6–47. https://doi.org/10.1037/a0038147

Ascarelli, M. (2010). *Independent vision: Dorothy Harrison Eustis and the story of the seeing eye*. Purdue University Press.

Banks, J. B., McCoy, C., & Trzcinski, C. (2018). Examining the impact of a brief human-canine interaction on stress and attention. *Human-Animal Interaction Bulletin*. https://doi.org/10.1079/hai.2018.0003

Barker, S. B., & Gee, N. R. (2021). Canine-assisted interventions in hospitals: Best practices for maximizing human and canine safety. *Frontiers in Veterinary Science*, 8, 1–12. https://doi.org/10.3389/fvets.2021.615730

Barker, S. B., Barker, R. T., McCain, N. L., & Schubert, C. M. (2016). A randomized cross-over exploratory study of the effect of visiting therapy dogs on college student stress before final exams. *Anthrozoös*, 29(1), 35–46. https://doi.org/10.1080/08927936.2015.1069988

Beck, A. M. (2014). The biology of the human–animal bond. *Animal Frontiers*, 4(3), 32–36. https://doi.org/10.2527/af.2014-0019

Beck, A. M., & Katcher, A. H. (1996). *Between pets and people: The importance of animal companionship*. Purdue University Press.

Beck, A. M., Barker, S., Gee, N. R., Griffin, J. A., & Johnson, R. (2018). The background to human-animal interaction (HAI) research. *Human-Animal Interaction Bulletin*. https://doi.org/10.1079/hai.2018.0015

Beetz, A., Kotrschal, K., Turner, D. C., Hediger, K., Uvnäs-Moberg, K., & Julius, H. (2011). The effect of a real dog, toy dog and friendly person on insecurely attached children during a stressful task: An exploratory study. *Anthrozoös*, 24(4), 349–368. https://doi.org/10.2752/175303711x13159027359746

Binfet, J. T. (2017). The effects of group-administered canine therapy on university students' wellbeing: A randomized controlled trial. *Anthrozoös*, 30(3), 397–414. https://doi.org/10.1080/08927936.2017.1335097

Binfet, J. T., & Hartwig, E. K. (2020). *Canine-assisted interventions: A comprehensive guide to credentialing therapy dog teams*. Routledge.

Binfet, J. T., & Passmore, H.-A. (2016). Hounds and homesickness: The effects of an animal-assisted therapeutic intervention for first-year university students. *Anthrozoös*, 29(3), 441–454. https://doi.org/10.1080/08927936.2016.1181364

Binfet, J. T., Green, F. L., & Draper, Z. A. (2021). The importance of client–canine contact in canine-assisted interventions: A randomized controlled trial. *Anthrozoös*, 35(1), 1–22. https://doi.org/10.1080/08927936.2021.1944558

Binfet, J. T., Passmore, H.-A., Cebry, A., Struik, K., & McKay, C. (2018). Reducing university students' stress through a drop-in canine-therapy program. *Journal of Mental Health*, 27(3), 197–204. https://doi.org/10.1080/09638237.2017.1417551

Bowlby, J. (1969). *Attachment and loss* (Vol. 1). Basic Books.

Braun, C., Stangler, T., Narveson, J., & Pettingell, S. (2009). Animal-assisted therapy as a pain relief intervention for children. *Complementary Therapies in Clinical Practice*, 15(2), 105–109. https://doi.org/10.1016/j.ctcp.2009.02.008

Burrows, K. E., Adams, C. L., & Spiers, J. (2008). Sentinels of safety: Service dogs ensure safety and enhance freedom and well-being for families with autistic children. *Qualitative Health Research*, 18(12), 1642–1649. https://doi.org/10.1177/1049732308327088

Carlisle, G. K. (2014). The social skills and attachment to dogs of children with autism spectrum disorder. *Journal of Autism and Developmental Disorders*, 45(5), 1137–1145. https://doi.org/10.1007/s10803-014-2267-7

Chalmers, D., & Dell, C. A. (2015). Applying one health to the study of animal-assisted interventions. *EcoHealth*, 12(4), 560–562. https://doi.org/10.1007/s10393-015-1042-3

Cobb, S. (1976). Social support as a moderator of life stress. *Psychosomatic Medicine*, 38(5), 300–314. https://doi.org/10.1097/00006842-197609000-00003

Cohen, S., & Wills, T. A. (1985). Stress, social support, and the buffering hypothesis. *Psychological Bulletin*, 98(2), 310–357. https://doi.org/10.1037/0033-2909.98.2.310

Corson, S. A., Arnold, L. E., Gwynne, P. H., & Corson, E. O. (1977). Pet dogs as nonverbal communication links in hospital psychiatry. *Comprehensive Psychiatry*, 18(1), 61–72. https://doi.org/10.1016/s0010-440x(77)80008-4

Crossman, M. K., Kazdin, A. E., & Knudson, K. (2015). Brief unstructured interaction with a dog reduces distress. *Anthrozoös*, 28(4), 649–659. https://doi.org/10.1080/08927936.2015.1070008

Crossman, M. K., Kazdin, A. E., Matijczak, A., Kitt, E. R., & Santos, L. R. (2020). The influence of interactions with dogs on affect, anxiety, and arousal in children. *Journal of Clinical Child & Adolescent Psychology*, 49(4), 535–548. https://doi.org/10.1080/15374416.2018.1520119

Eddy, J., Hart, L. A., & Boltz, R. P. (2001). The effects of service dogs on social acknowledgments of people in wheelchairs. *The Journal of Psychology*, 122(1), 39–45. https://doi.org/10.1080/00223980.1988.10542941

Fine, A. H. (2014). *Our faithful companions: Exploring the essence of our kinship with animals.* Alpine.

Fine, A. H., & Ferrell, J. (2021). Conceptualizing the human–animal bond and animal-assisted interventions. *The Welfare of Animals in Animal-Assisted Interventions*, (1), 21–41. https://doi.org/10.1007/978-3-030-69587-3_2

Fine, A. H., & Chastain Griffin, T. (2022). Protecting animal welfare in animal-assisted intervention: Our ethical obligation. *Seminars in Speech and Language*, 43(01), 8–23. https://doi.org/10.1055/s-0041-1742099

Fine, A. H., & Weaver, S. J. (2018). The human–animal bond and animal-assisted intervention. *Oxford Textbook of Nature and Public Health*, 132–138. https://doi.org/10.1093/med/9780198725916.003.0028

Fine, A. H., Mueller, M. K., Ng, Z. Y., Beck, A. M., & Peralta, J. M. (2023). *The Routledge international handbook of human-animal interactions and anthrozoology.* Routledge.

Fine, A., Beck, A., & Ng, Z. (2019). The state of animal-assisted interventions: Addressing the contemporary issues that will shape the future. *International Journal of Environmental Research and Public Health*, 16(20), 3997. https://doi.org/10.3390/ijerph16203997

Gee, N. R., & Mueller, M. K. (2019). A systematic review of research on pet ownership and Animal Interactions among older adults. *Anthrozoös*, 32(2), 183–207. https://doi.org/10.1080/08927936.2019.1569903

Gee, N. R., Fine, A. H., & Schuck, S. (2015). Animals in educational settings: Research and practice. In A. H. Fine (Ed.), *Handbook on animal-assisted therapy: Foundations and guidelines for animal-assisted interventions* (4th ed., pp. 195–210). Elsevier Academic Press. https://doi.org/10.1016/B978-0-12-801292-5.00014-6

Gee, N. R., Griffin, J. A., & McCardle, P. (2017). Human–animal interaction research in school settings: Current knowledge and future directions. *AERA Open*, 3(3), 1–9. https://doi.org/10.1177/2332858417724346

Gee, N. R., Rodriguez, K. E., Fine, A. H., & Trammell, J. P. (2021). Dogs supporting human health and well-being: A biopsychosocial approach. *Frontiers in Veterinary Science*, 8, 1–11. https://doi.org/10.3389/fvets.2021.630465

Grajfoner, D., Harte, E., Potter, L., & McGuigan, N. (2017).The effect of dog-assisted intervention on student well-being, mood, and anxiety. *International Journal of Environmental Research and Public Health*, 14(5), 483. https://doi.org/10.3390/ijerph14050483

Guest, C. M. (2006). Hearing dogs: A longitudinal study of social and psychological effects on deaf and hard-of-hearing recipients. *Journal of Deaf Studies and Deaf Education*, 11(2), 252–261. https://doi.org/10.1093/deafed/enj028

Hall, S. S., Gee, N. R., & Mills, D. S. (2016). Children reading to dogs: A systematic review of the literature. *PLOS ONE*, 11(2). https://doi.org/10.1371/journal.pone.0149759

Handlin, L., Hydbring-Sandberg, E., Nilsson, A., Ejdebäck, M., Jansson, A., & Uvnäs-Moberg, K. (2011). Short-term interaction between dogs and their owners: Effects on oxytocin, cortisol, insulin and heart rate—an exploratory study. *Anthrozoös*, 24(3), 301–315. https://doi.org/10.2752/175303711x13045914865385

Haraway, D. J. (2008). *When species meet*. University of Minnesota Press.

Hediger, K., & Turner, D. C. (2014). Can dogs increase children's attention and concentration performance? A randomised controlled trial. *Human-Animal Interaction Bulletin*, 2(3), 21–39. https://doi.org/10.1079/hai.2014.0010

Howell, T. J., Nieforth, L., Thomas-Pino, C., Samet, L., Agbonika, S., Cuevas-Pavincich, F., Fry, N. E., Hill, K., Jegatheesan, B., Kakinuma, M., MacNamara, M., Mattila-Rautiainen, S., Perry, A., Tardif-Williams, C. Y., Walsh, E. A., Winkle, M., Yamamoto, M., Yerbury, R., Rawat, V., … Bennett, P. (2022). Defining terms used for animals working in support roles for people with support needs. *Animals*, 12(15), 1975. https://doi.org/10.3390/ani12151975

Hunt, M. G., & Chizkov, R. R. (2014). Are therapy dogs like xanax? Does animal-assisted therapy impact processes relevant to cognitive behavioral psychotherapy? *Anthrozoös*, 27(3), 457–469. https://doi.org/10.2752/175303714x14023922797959

Hupcey, J. E. (1998). Social support: Assessing conceptual coherence. *Qualitative Health Research*, 8(3), 304–318. https://doi.org/10.1177/104973239800800302

International Association of Human-Animal Interaction Organizations. (2018). *The IAHAIO definitions for animal assisted intervention and guidelines for wellness of animals involved in AAI* [White paper]. IAHAIO. https://iahaio.org/best-practice/white-paper-on-animal-assisted-interventions/

Janssens, M., Janssens, E., Eshuis, J., Lataster, J., Simons, M., Reijnders, J., & Jacobs, N. (2021). Companion animals as buffer against the impact of stress on affect: An experience sampling study. *Animals*, 11(8), 2171. https://doi.org/10.3390/ani11082171

Jegatheesan, B., Beetz, A., Ormerod, E., Johnson, R., Fine, A., Yamazaki, K., Dudzik, C., Maria Garcia, R., Winkle, M., & Choi, G. (2014). *IAHAIO white paper 2014*. IAHAIO. https://iahaio.org/wp/wp-content/uploads/2017/05/iahaio-white-paper-final-nov-24-2014.pdf

Julius, H., Beetz, A., Kotrschal, K., Turner, D., Uvnas-Moberg, K., & Matamonasa-Bennett, A. (2013). Book review: "Attachment to pets: An integrative view of human-animal relationships for therapeutic practice" (2013). *Human-Animal Interaction Bulletin*. https://doi.org/10.1079/hai.2013.0009

Katayama, M., Kubo, T., Yamakawa, T., Fujiwara, K., Nomoto, K., Ikeda, K., Mogi, K., Nagasawa, M., & Kikusui, T. (2019). Emotional contagion from humans to dogs is facilitated by duration of ownership. *Frontiers in Psychology*, 10, 1–11. https://doi.org/10.3389/fpsyg.2019.01678

Kellert, S. R., & Wilson, E. O. (1993). *The biophilia hypothesis*. Island Press.

Kline, J. A., Fisher, M. A., Pettit, K. L., Linville, C. T., & Beck, A. M. (2019). Controlled clinical trial of canine therapy versus usual care to reduce patient anxiety in the emergency department. *PLOS ONE*, 14(1). https://doi.org/10.1371/journal.pone.0209232

Krause-Parello, C. A., & Friedmann, E. (2014). The effects of an animal-assisted intervention on salivary alpha-amylase, salivary immunoglobulin A, and heart rate during forensic interviews in child sexual abuse cases. *Anthrozoös*, 27(4), 581–590. https://doi.org/10.2752/089279314x14072268688005

Kruger, K. A., & Serpell, J. A. (2006). Animal-assisted interventions in mental health: Definitions and theoretical foundations. In A. H. Fine (Ed.), *Handbook on animal-assisted therapy: Theoretical foundations and guidelines for practice* (pp. 21–38). Academic Press. https://doi.org/10.1016/b978-0-12-381453-1.10003-0

Kruger, K. A., & Serpell, J. A. (2010). Animal-assisted interventions in mental health: Definitions and theoretical foundations. *Handbook on Animal-Assisted Therapy*, 33–48. https://doi.org/10.1016/b978-0-12-381453-1.10003-0

Levinson, B. M. (1962). The dog as a "co-therapist." *Mental Hygiene*, 46, 59–65.

Levinson, B. M. (1969). *Pet-oriented child psychotherapy* (1st ed.). Charles C. Thomas.

Levinson, B. M. (1987). Foreword. In P. Arkow (Eds.), *The loving bond: Companion animals in the helping professions* (pp. 1–20). R & E Publishers.

Marcus, D. A. (2013). The science behind animal-assisted therapy. *Current Pain and Headache Reports*, 17(4), 322. https://doi.org/10.1007/s11916-013-0322-2

Matsuoka, A. K., & Sorenson, J. (2018). *Critical animal studies: Towards trans-species social justice*. Rowman & Littlefield International.

McBride, E. A., & Baugh, S. (2022). Animal welfare in context: Historical, scientific, ethical, moral and one welfare perspectives. In A. Vitale & S. Pollo (Eds.), *Human/animal relationships in transformation: Scientific, moral and legal perspectives* (pp. 119–147). The Palgrave Macmillan Animal Ethics Series.

Mission and goals. (n.d.). IAHAIO. Retrieved June 13, 2024, from https://iahaio.org/missions-goals/

Mission. (n.d.-a). American Humane. Retrieved June 14, 2024, from https://www.americanhumane.org/humane-heartland/mission/

Mission. (n.d.-b). International Society for Anthrozoology (ISAZ). Retrieved June 14, 2024, from https://isaz.net/who-we-are/

Mossello, E., Ridolfi, A., Mello, A. M., Lorenzini, G., Mugnai, F., Piccini, C., Barone, D., Peruzzi, A., Masotti, G., & Marchionni, N. (2011). Animal-assisted activity and emotional status of patients with alzheimer's disease in day care. *International Psychogeriatrics*, 23(6), 899–905. https://doi.org/10.1017/s1041610211000226

Mueller, M. K., Anderson, E. C., King, E. K., & Urry, H. L. (2021). Null effects of therapy dog interaction on adolescent anxiety during a laboratory-based social evaluative stressor. *Anxiety, Stress, & Coping: An International Journal*, 34(4), 365–380. https://doi.org/10.1080/10615806.2021.1892084

Nagasawa, M., Mitsui, S., En, S., Ohtani, N., Ohta, M., Sakuma, Y., Onaka, T., Mogi, K., & Kikusui, T. (2015). Oxytocin-gaze positive loop and the coevolution of human-dog bonds. *Science*, 348(6232), 333–336. https://doi.org/10.1126/science.1261022

Nagengast, S. L., Baun, M. M., Megel, M., & Michael Leibowitz, J. (1997). The effects of the presence of a companion animal on physiological arousal and behavioral distress in children during a physical examination. *Journal of Pediatric Nursing*, 12(6), 323–330. https://doi.org/10.1016/s0882-5963(97)80058-9

Ng, Z., Albright, J., Fine, A. H., & Peralta, J. (2015). Our ethical and moral responsibility: Ensuring the welfare of therapy animals. In A. H. Fine (Ed.), *Handbook on animal-assisted therapy: Foundations and guidelines for animal-assisted interventions* (4th ed., pp. 91–101). Academic Press/Elsevier.

Nimer, J., & Lundahl, B. (2007). Animal-assisted therapy: A meta-analysis. *Anthrozoös*, 20(3), 225–238. https://doi.org/10.2752/089279307x224773

O'Haire, M. (2010). Companion animals and human health: Benefits, challenges, and the road ahead. *Journal of Veterinary Behavior*, 5(5), 226–234. https://doi.org/10.1016/j.jveb.2010.02.002

Odendaal, J. S. J., & Meintjes, R. A. (2003). Neurophysiological correlates of affiliative behaviour between humans and dogs. *The Veterinary Journal*, 165(3), 296–301. https://doi.org/10.1016/s1090-0233(02)00237-x

Our Story. (n.d.). Therapeutic Paws of Canada (TPOC). Retrieved June 14, 2024, from https://tpoc.ca/our-story/

Parbery-Clark, C., Lubamba, M., Tanner, L., & McColl, E. (2021). Animal-assisted interventions for the improvement of mental health outcomes in higher education students: A systematic review of randomised controlled trials. *International Journal of Environmental Research and Public Health*, 18(20), 10768. https://doi.org/10.3390/ijerph182010768

Payne, E., Bennett, P., & McGreevy, P. (2015). Current perspectives on attachment and bonding in the dog and human dyad. *Psychology Research and Behavior Management*, 8, 71–79. https://doi.org/10.2147/prbm.s74972

Pendry, P., & Vandagriff, J. L. (2019). Animal Visitation Program (AVP) reduces cortisol levels of university students: A randomized controlled trial. *AERA Open*, 5(2). https://doi.org/10.1177/2332858419852592

Pendry, P., Carr, A. M., Roeter, S. M., & Vandagriff, J. L. (2018). Experimental trial demonstrates effects of animal-assisted stress prevention program on college students' positive and negative emotion. *Human-Animal Interaction Bulletin*, 6, 81–97. https://doi.org/10.1079/hai.2018.0004

Peralta, J. M., & Fine, A. H. (2021). *The welfare of animals in animal-assisted interventions: Foundations and best practice methods*. Springer.

Pinillos, R. G. (2018). The path to developing a one welfare framework. *One Welfare: A Framework to Improve Animal Welfare and Human Well-Being*, 1–15. https://doi.org/10.1079/9781786393845.0001

Rault, J.-L., van den Munkhof, M., & Buisman-Pijlman, F. T. (2017). Oxytocin as an indicator of psychological and social well-being in domesticated animals: A critical review. *Frontiers in Psychology*, 8. https://doi.org/10.3389/fpsyg.2017.01521

Reilly, K. M., Adesope, O. O., & Erdman, P. (2020). The effects of dogs on learning: A meta-analysis. *Anthrozoös*, 33(3), 339–360. https://doi.org/10.1080/08927936.2020.1746523

Sable, P. (1995). Pets, attachment, and well-being across the life cycle. *Social Work*, 40(3), 334–341. https://doi.org/10.1093/sw/40.3.334

Sandt, D. D. (2020). Effective implementation of animal assisted education interventions in the inclusive early childhood education classroom. *Early Childhood Education Journal*, 48(1), 103–115. https://doi.org/10.1007/s10643-019-01000-z

Santaniello, A., Dicé, F., Claudia Carratú, R., Amato, A., Fioretti, A., & Menna, L. F. (2020). Methodological and terminological issues in animal-assisted interventions: An umbrella review of systematic reviews. *Animals*, 10(5), 759. https://doi.org/10.3390/ani10050759

Schaefer, C., Coyne, J. C., & Lazarus, R. S. (1981). The health-related functions of social support. *Journal of Behavioral Medicine*, 4(4), 381–406. https://doi.org/10.1007/bf00846149

Schuck, S. E., & Fine, A. H. (2017). School-based animal-assisted interventions for children with deficits in executive function. *How Animals Help Students Learn*, 69–82. https://doi.org/10.4324/9781315620619-6

Schuck, S. E., Emmerson, N. A., Fine, A. H., & Lakes, K. D. (2015). Canine-assisted therapy for children with ADHD: Preliminary findings from the positive assertive cooperative kids study. *Journal of Attention Disorders*, 19(2), 125–137. https://doi.org/10.1177/1087054713502080

Serpell, J. (1996). *In the company of animals: A study of human-animal relationships*. Cambridge University Press.

Shapiro, K. (2020). Human-animal studies: Remembering the past, celebrating the present, troubling the future. *Society & Animals*, 28(7), 797–833. https://doi.org/10.1163/15685306-bja10029

Sirovica, L. V., & Keyserlingk, M. A. G. (2023). Public perceptions of farm animal welfare. *The Routledge International Handbook of Human-Animal Interactions and Anthrozoology*, 644–657. https://doi.org/10.4324/9781032153346-44

Therapy dog program. (2024). St. John Ambulance. Retrieved June 14, 2024, from https://www.sja.ca/en/community-services/therapy-dog-program

Thielke, L. E., & Udell, M. A. R. (2020). Characterizing human–dog attachment relationships in foster and shelter environments as a potential mechanism for achieving mutual wellbeing and success. *Animals*, 10(1), 67. https://doi.org/10.3390/ani10010067

Travers, C., Perkins, J., Rand, J., Bartlett, H., & Morton, J. (2013). An evaluation of dog-assisted therapy for residents of aged care facilities with dementia. *Anthrozoös*, 26(2), 213–225. https://doi.org/10.2752/175303713x13636846944169

Trevathan-Minnis, M., Schroeder, K., & Eccles, E. (2023). Changing with the times: A qualitative content analysis of perceptions toward the study and practice of human–animal interactions. *The Humanistic Psychologist*, 51(2), 150–159. https://doi.org/10.1037/hum0000251

Tsai, C. C., Friedmann, E., & Thomas, S. A. (2010). The effect of animal-assisted therapy on stress responses in hospitalized children. *Anthrozoös*, 23(3), 245–258. https://doi.org/10.2752/175303710X12750451258977

Viau, R., Arsenault-Lapierre, G., Fecteau, S., Champagne, N., Walker, C.-D., & Lupien, S. (2010). Effect of service dogs on salivary cortisol secretion in autistic children. *Psychoneuroendocrinology*, 35(8), 1187–1193. https://doi.org/10.1016/j.psyneuen.2010.02.004

von Keyserlingk, M. A. G., & Weary, D. M. (2017). A 100-year review: Animal welfare in the Journal of Dairy Science—the first 100 years. *Journal of Dairy Science*, 100(12), 10432–10444. https://doi.org/10.3168/jds.2017-13298

Ward-Griffin, E., Klaiber, P., Collins, H. K., Owens, R. L., Coren, S., & Chen, F. S. (2018). Petting away pre-exam stress: The effect of therapy dog sessions on student well-being. *Stress and Health*, 34(3), 468–473. https://doi.org/10.1002/smi.2804

Wilks, S. E., & Spivey, C. A. (2010). Resilience in undergraduate social work students: Social support and adjustment to academic stress1. *Social Work Education*, 29(3), 276–288. https://doi.org/10.1080/02615470902912243

Wilson, E. O. (1984). *Biophilia*. Harvard University Press.

Winkle, M., & Johnson Binder, A. (2024). The importance of animal welfare in animal-assisted services. *Animal Behaviour and Welfare Cases*, 1–4. https://doi.org/10.1079/abwcases.2024.0003

Wohlfarth, R., Mutschler, B., Beetz, A., Kreuser, F., & Korsten-Reck, U. (2013). Dogs motivate obese children for physical activity: Key elements of a motivational theory of animal-assisted interventions. *Frontiers in Psychology*, 4. https://doi.org/10.3389/fpsyg.2013.00796

Wood, E., Ohlsen, S., Thompson, J., Hulin, J., & Knowles, L. (2017). The feasibility of brief dog-assisted therapy on university students stress levels: The paws study. *Journal of Mental Health*, 27(3), 263–268. https://doi.org/10.1080/09638237.2017.1385737

Wright, H., Hall, S., Hames, A., Hardiman, J., Mills, R., PAWS Project Team, & Mills, D. (2015). Pet dogs improve family functioning and reduce anxiety in children with autism spectrum disorder. *Anthrozoös*, 28(4), 611–624. https://doi.org/10.1080/08927936.2015.1070003

APPENDIX 2.1

Illustrations of Animal Therapy Organizations Around the World

Animal Therapy
Organizations Around The World

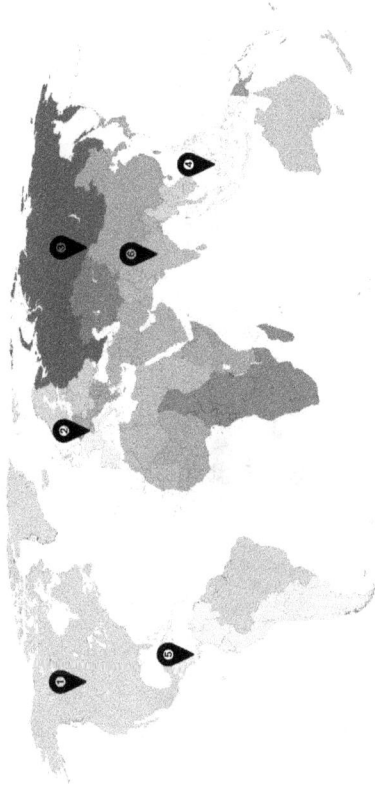

Please note that this is not an extensive list. Please visit the IAHAIO for more

North America
Canada
United States

North & Western Europe
Austria
France
Germany
Portugal
United Kingdom

Central & Eastern
Europe & Central Asia
Czech Republic
Turkey

East, Southeast Asia, & Pacific
Australia
China
Japan
New Zealand
Singapore

Latin America & Caribbean
Mexico

South Asia
India

❶ North America

Canada

- 1982 - BC Pets and Friends
https://www.petsandfriends.org/about/
- 1992 - St. John Ambulance Therapy Dog Program
https://sja.ca/en/community-services/therapy-dog-program ;
https://m.subaru.ca/WebPage.aspx?WebSiteID=282&WebPage
ID=21370
- 1996 - National Service Dogs
https://nsd.on.ca
- 1998 - The Canadian Foundation for Animal-Assisted Support
Services
https://www.cf4aass.ca
- 2002 - Therapeutic Paws of Canada
https://tpoc.ca
- 2012 - Wounded Warriors Canada
https://woundedwarriors.ca

United States

- 1945 - American Humane
https://www.americanhumane.org/humane-
heartland/mission/
- 1976 - Therapy Dogs International
https://www.tdi-dog.org/default.aspx
- 1977 - Pet Partners
https://petpartners.org
- 1979 - The Center for the Interaction of Animals and Society
https://core.ac.uk/download/pdf/214149868.pdf

- 1983 - Canine Companions for Independence
https://rarediseases.org/organizations/canine-companions-for-
independence/
- 1986 - Assistance Dogs International
https://assistancedogsinternational.org
- 1988 - The Good Dog Foundation
https://thegooddogfoundation.org/about-us/#mission
- 1988 - Therapaws of Michigan
https://therapaws.org
- 1991 - Canine Therapy Corps
https://www.caninetherapycorps.org
- 1992 - International Association of Human-Animal Interaction
Organizations
https://iahaio.org/missions-goals/
- 1994 - Alliance of Therapy Dogs
https://www.therapydogs.com
- 1995 - Love on a Leash
https://www.loveonaleash.org
- 1999 - Bright & Beautiful Therapy Dogs
https://golden-dogs.org/contact/
- 2005 - Paws for People
https://www.pawsforpeople.org/aboutus/
- 2008 - Therapy Dogs United
https://www.therapydogsunited.org/about/
- 2010 - Animal Assisted Therapy Programs of Colorado
https://www.animalassistedtherapyprograms.org
- Unknown - Human-Animal Interaction: APA Division 17,
Section 13
https://www.human-animal-interaction.org

❷ Northern & Western Europe

Austria
- Akademie Tiergestützt
https://www.akademie-tiergestuetzt.com

France
- 1971 - Adrienne and Pierre Sommer Foundation
https://fondation-apsommer.org

Germany
- Animal Advocate e.V. TTA-NRW
https://tta-nrw.de

Portugal
- 2002 - Animals
https://animasportugal.org/animas/

United Kingdom
- 1979 - Five Freedoms
https://webarchive.nationalarchives.gov.uk/ukgwa/201210100
12427/http://www.fawc.org.uk/freedoms.htm
- 1979 - Society of Companion Animal Studies
http://www.scas.org.uk/about/
- 1983 - Pets As Therapy
https://petsastherapy.org/information/about-us
- 1988 - Canine Concerns Scotland Trust
https://www.therapet.org.uk
- 1990 - International Society for Anthrozoology
https://isaz.net

- 2006 - International Society for Animal Assisted Therapy
https://isaat.org
- 2013 - Animal Assisted Intervention International
https://aai-int.org
- 2016 - Therapy Dogs Nationwide
https://tdn.org.uk

❸ Central & Eastern Europe & Central Asia

Czech Republic
- 2001 - Canistherapy Training Association Hafik
https://www.canisterapie.org/about-us

Turkey
- Unknown - Center for Education, Animal Assisted
Interventions & Green Care
https://www.cac-greencare.com

❹ East, Southeast Asia, & Pacific

Australia
- 1996 - Assistance Dogs Australia
https://www.assistancedogs.org.au
- 2012 - Centre for Service and Therapy Dogs Australia
https://www.cstda.com.au
- 2015 - Cherished Pets
https://www.cherishedpetcare.com.au/foundation/about-
foundation

57 **History of Canine-Assisted Interventions**

•Unknown - Therapy Dogs Australia
https://therapydog.com.au
•Unknown - Therapy Animals Australia
https://therapyanimals.com.au/about/
•Unknown - Canine Comprehension
https://www.caninecomprehension.com.au

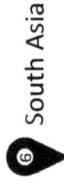

China
•1991 - Animals Asia - Dr. Dogs
https://www.animalsasia.org/us/our-work/cat-and-dog-welfare/what-we-do/dr-dog.html

Japan
•Unknown - International Therapy Dog Association
https://therapydog-a.org/en/organization/
https://okinawa.therapydog-a.org

New Zealand
•2018 - Therapy Dogs New Zealand
https://therapydogs.co.nz

Singapore
•Unknown - Animal-Assisted Interactions Singapore
https://aai.sg

⑤ Latin America & Caribbean

Mexico
•Unknown - ApapáchaDogs A.C.
https://apapacha.me

⑥ South Asia

India
•2003 - Animal Angels Foundation
https://animalangels.org.in

Three

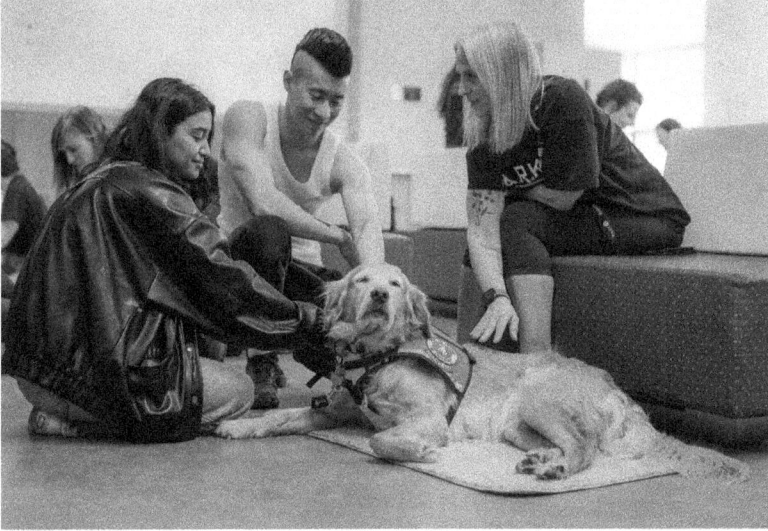

Figure 3.1 Volunteer handler Eirena provides guidance to facilitate an interaction between her therapy dog Baylee and two undergraduate students

Source: F. L. L. Green Photography; used with permission

DOI: 10.4324/9781032639284-3

SCENARIO

Therapy Dogs Who Are Settled Themselves Settle Excited Humans

> I can see you're excited to meet my dog Henry but I'm going to ask you to stop and take a deep breath before you approach. Henry's job is to help you feel less stressed and that's tough to do when you're really excited.

As part of her handler orientation and training with her therapy dog organization, Liz was taught that she was in control of, and was to oversee, the interactions between her dog and members of the public, and when she was asked to participate in a local high school's Mental Health Week activities, she knew she'd encounter students whose enthusiasm ran high. She knew she couldn't be too stern with her instructions or she'd discourage the interaction but she also knew she had to convey that a calm approach to meeting her dog was in everyone's best interest. As the student took out her phone to take a photo, Liz said, "We'll have time for photos but let me first introduce you to my dog and get his approval for you two to interact. This is Henry and he likes to be petted this way. Let me show you."

QUESTIONS FOR REFLECTION

1. What information or instructions should a handler provide to visiting clients?

2. What are the emotions that visiting clients might bring to an interaction?

3. What is the handler's role in safeguarding the welfare of their therapy dog?

4. How might a handler redirect an overly excited visitor?

5. How can visitors to a session optimize their interaction with a therapy dog?

These instructions from a handler to an approaching high school student illustrate the role of the handler in overseeing the interaction between their dog and a visiting client, providing instruction to the client around behavioural expectations, and how handlers work to safeguard their dog's welfare. In the scenario featured here, a teen excitedly rushing up to greet a dog runs the risk of startling the dog and a more measured approach and introduction helps ensure that the interaction respects and supports dog welfare. In particular, we see the handler ask the client to calibrate their energy or excitement by taking a deep breath. In doing so, the handler ensures that the client manages their emotions and energy prior to interacting (Figure 3.1).

The aim of this chapter is to explore, in depth, the welfare of dog-handler teams. Here we build upon the definition of welfare proffered in Chapter 1 and define welfare as it pertains to the dog and the handler, examine the responsibilities of varied agents in safeguarding welfare, explore the emotional synergy between handlers and dogs with respect to welfare, and examine research exploring dog-handler team welfare.

EXTENDING AND DEEPENING OUR DEFINITION OF DOG-HANDLER TEAM WELFARE

In our opening chapter, we introduced an overarching definition of animal welfare by leveraging Ng and colleagues' (2015, p. 359) definition:

> Very good welfare and well-being status is characterized by a state in which an animal is free from distress most of the time, is in good physical health, exhibits a substantial range of species-specific behaviors, and is able to cope effectively with environmental stimuli.
>
> (Hetts et al., 1992; Novak & Drewsen, 1989)

As the above definition of welfare is intended for animals more broadly, we see the need to more specifically define welfare for therapy dogs working within the context of CAIs. We also acknowledged in Chapter 1 that absent from the broad definition of animal welfare was the notion of consent, and in our definition below, we situate consent at the heart of our interpretation of welfare. By seeking consent with a lowered open palm facing upwards, the visiting client is asking for permission to interact. Doing so allows the dog to acknowledge the visitor, to sniff their hand, and to offer their consent or agreement to continue interacting (Figures 3.2 and 3.3).

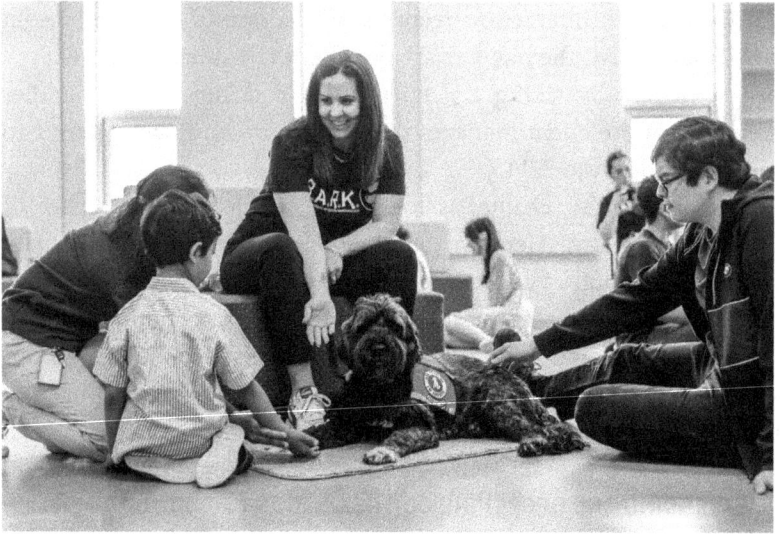

Figure 3.2 Handler Kimberly demonstrates to a young child how to position the hand to obtain dog consent prior to interacting. Her therapy dog, Patrick, waits patiently in a lie down position
Source: F. L. L. Green Photography; used with permission

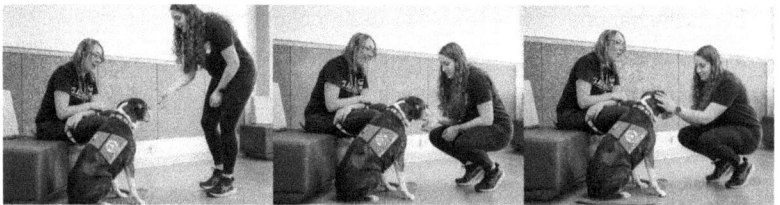

Figure 3.3 Sequence of obtaining consent from a dog. Karen, an undergraduate student, approaches handler Michelle and therapy dog Maya slowly and offers her hand to obtain consent prior to petting Maya gently. Maya sits on her comfort mat facing Karen.
Source: F. L. L. Green Photography; used with permission

Incorporating the practice of obtaining consent into a definition of therapy dog welfare as a part of CAIs allows us to proffer the following definition of therapy dog welfare:

> Therapy dog welfare within a CAI is a state of well-being monitored and facilitated by a handler who sees the dog consent to an interaction with a human, demonstrates behaviours reflecting that the interaction is welcomed (e.g., prompting the human for additional petting, leaning into client, etc.), demonstrates behaviour free of agitation or distress (i.e., excessive panting, shaking, whale eye, etc.), and where the dog has the freedom to retreat from the interaction of their own freewill (i.e., not crowded and with a pathway to retreat) without negative consequences (i.e., redirection or correction from handler).

Embedded within our definition of therapy dog welfare, we see key elements highlighted that include identifying the roles/responsibilities of the handler, positioning consent at the outset of the process, recognizing dog behaviour as an indicator or barometer of emotional and physical well-being and an emphasis on dog agency and enjoyment, and the importance of providing a retreat pathway to cease the interaction.

Moving Beyond Therapy Dogs Tolerating Interactions

In offering the above definition of therapy dog welfare, we recognize that welfare is measured in degrees and can shift, change, and vary. Welfare quality might be described by descriptors on a continuum of *low*, *medium*, and *high*. That is, it is not merely present or absent. Rather, welfare is a fluid condition or state *within* and *over the course of* a CAI. It requires constant monitoring by the handler and program personnel and may require adaptations or modifications on the part of the handler or program staff. This might see a handler cue or prompt a dog to alert them to an approaching client or when program personnel restrict the number of clients within a session to prevent overcrowding. This constant monitoring of therapy dog welfare helps ensure that interacting with humans is, and remains, enjoyable for the dog. In our opening scenario, we saw evidence of the handler monitoring the initial approach of an excited high school student – to temper the interaction and to help create conditions in which an optimal human-animal interaction might occur.

Dogs' Abilities to Regulate Stress within Sessions

A curious point regarding therapy dogs and indicators of stress is raised in a recent paper by Clark and colleagues (2020) who, in a pilot study of nine dog-handler teams working to support patients in a hospital context, measured stress in both therapy dogs and handlers. They did this in two distinct ways: (1) by measuring cortisol and (2) through self-perceptions of handler stress and observations of therapy dog stress. Their findings revealed that dog and handler stress did not increase over the course of visits with clients and that handlers were perceptive of the indicators reflecting their dog's welfare. As observations to identify stress indicators in therapy dogs were a part of the methodology used in this study, these authors highlight that some stress indicators (e.g., shaking, lip licking) may be reflective of dogs *coping* with or *adapting* to stress arising within sessions. That is, to the outside observer, such behaviours could be interpreted as signs of stress however they could be a means through which the dogs manage or reduce feeling stressed – how they adjust to and adapt to the stimuli they encounter. In this regard, these behaviours should be encouraged as they help the dog regulate the stress they're experiencing. This might be akin to a human doing a neck roll or wringing their hands to alleviate nervousness. But how might one distinguish between coping behaviours and behaviours more directly indicative of the dog experiencing stress? This is certainly a grey area, and although this notion of coping behaviours to address stress has been raised in research with agility dogs (Pastore et al., 2011) and shelter dogs (Shiverdecker et al., 2013), an extant review of the literature identifies this as an understudied topic vis-à-vis therapy dogs. In our last chapter (Chapter 8), we'll raise this as an area warranting additional research.

The Importance of Building Therapy Dog's Capacity Over Time

A therapy dog's ability to withstand the stressors inherent in participating in CAIs can be enhanced by building the dog's capacity incrementally over time. After successfully passing an organization's assessment and evaluation protocols, program personnel are wise to schedule dog-handler teams for short, abbreviated sessions rather

Table 3.1 Stimuli Encountered by a Therapy Dog When Working in a CAI

New location	Flooring
New building	Comfort mat (if provided)
Working space where CAI held (isolated room or shared space?)	Spacing between other dog-handler teams
Temperature of room	Volume of visitors to station
Greeting by organization personnel	Diversity and needs of visitors (e.g., wheelchairs, variability in clothing, etc.)
Other dog and handler teams in shared space	Wearing therapy dog identification (e.g., vest or scarf)
Multiple greetings by visiting clients	Odours (e.g., food nearby)
Varied emotions presented by clients	Repeated touch by clients
Emotional state of handler	Unfamiliar water bowl
Unfamiliar noise (e.g., machinery, public announcements)	Stretch or bathroom breaks if offered and re-entering working space

than immediately asking the team to attend full-length sessions. After several successful short sessions, teams may then be asked to attend regular programming, but rushing dogs through to full participation too quickly risks them poorly adapting to the demands of engaging in sessions.

Related to the above, briefly consider all the stimuli that therapy dogs must adapt to when working in CAIs, keeping in mind that dogs don't always work in the same location in support of the same client. We offer this preliminary list to invite initial reflection around the varied stimuli encountered by therapy dogs; we will explore, in depth, additional stimuli in Chapter 5 (Table 3.1).

In examining the characteristics of handlers in Chapter 1, we introduced readers to animal-assisted crisis response (AACR; Eaton-Stull et al., 2023) dog-handler teams. Recall these are dog-handler teams who provide support to individuals who've experienced a disaster or crisis. As an illustration of the adaptability and resiliency of therapy dogs as well as the expectations of AACR dogs, consider the complexities inherent in the description by Eaton-Stull et al. (2023, p. 2):

Dogs providing AACR should be friendly, calm, obedient, and healthy. Accordingto Chandler (2012), not all dogs are suitable for AACR, and they have to be highlytolerant and non-reactive to stress, chaos, and noise. Most importantly, they mustbe reliable and respond consistently to commands. Dogs should be trained to usedifferent modes of transportation and maintain composure even when strange smells, sights, and sounds appear.

(Stewart et al., 2016)

Germane to our discussion and the overall mandate of our book, we would be remiss if we did not acknowledge Eaton-Stull and colleague's commitment to welfare. They write, "... handlers must be aware of their canine partners' stress and fatigue indicators, especially during deployment, and intervene accordingly before letting the dog surpass stress levels" (Lackey & Haberstock, 2019).

WELFARE – A DISTRIBUTED AND SHARED RESPONSIBILITY

Safeguarding the welfare of dog-handler teams is the shared responsibility of all the agents involved in the organization, delivery, and oversight of CAIs. This responsibility is shared by booking institutions, program personnel, handlers, and visiting clients. Collectively, when all agents uphold welfare standards, welfare is optimized for both dogs and handlers. We'll examine the responsibilities of each next (Figure 3.4).

Booking Institutions

Dog-handler teams are known to work in a variety of contexts in support of a variety of clients. This might include supporting children in a school seeking to strengthen their readings skills, law-enforcement personnel seeking a well-being break as part of their workday, or seniors in a retirement facility seeking to reduce feelings of isolation and loneliness (see Figure 3.5).

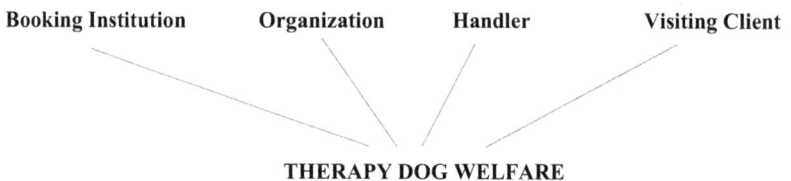

Figure 3.4 Varied agents in CAIs

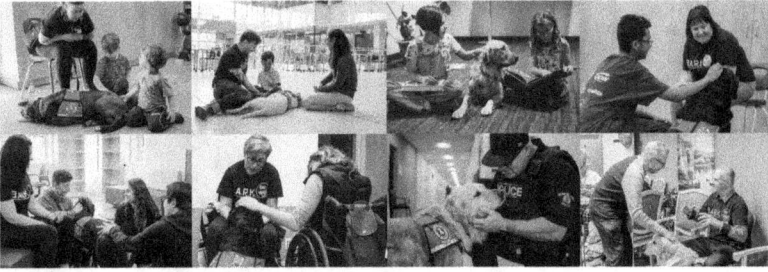

Figure 3.5 Illustrations of the variability of clients supported by therapy dogs
Source: Freya L. L. Green and Adam Lauzé Photography; used with permission

As a starting point, the institution that books the visit of dog-handler teams through a therapy dog organization should ideally identify a point-of-contact liaison who can meet the dog-handler team(s) upon their arrival, guide them to their working space, and ensure that adequate space is provided that will allow dog-handler teams to thrive and optimally work. This may be comprised of providing signage to notify all occupants of the building that dogs are present and working, communicating to the organization parking information for handlers and how best to enter and exit the building, providing protected space where dog-handler teams can set up and ensuring the temperature in the room is not too warm, ensuring no food is made available or served in the space, ensuring the floor has been cleaned to avoid dogs ingesting dropped food or medication, and having a janitorial plan in place to clean the space post-visit (see Figure 3.6).

Program Personnel

There is a plethora of organizations that organize, facilitate, and oversee opportunities for varied members of the public to interact with therapy dogs (recall the history of such organizations provided in Chapter 2 as well as the illustrations of programs worldwide at the end of this same chapter). The program personnel or the individuals responsible for overseeing the implementation of CAIs bear a responsibility to ensure that the conceptualization and application of therapy dog welfare is positioned front and centre in the organization's mission and vision. Doing so indicates that optimizing welfare is a priority, that resources are devoted to ensuring that welfare standards are

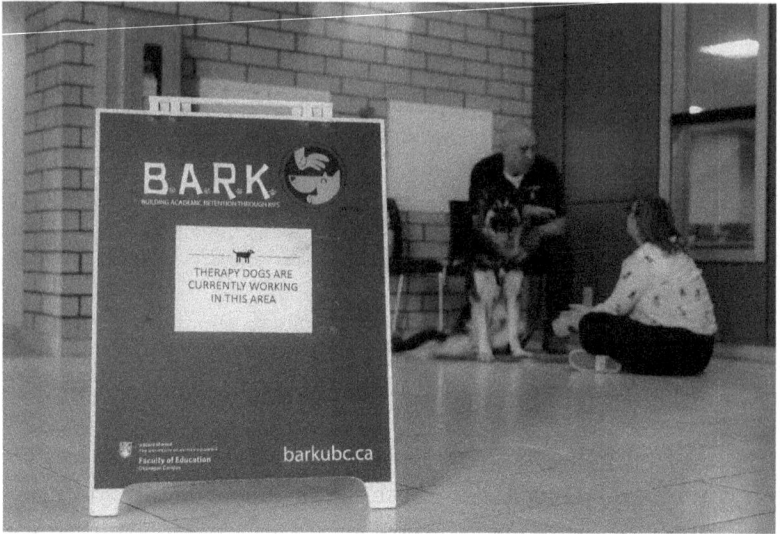

Figure 3.6 Signage notifying the public that dogs are working in an area. John-Tyler and Henry, a handler-therapy dog team, interact with an undergraduate student in the background
Source: Freya L. L. Green Photography; used with permission

met, and that handlers working in applied programming on behalf of the organization uphold these welfare standards. Further, program personnel bear the responsibility of monitoring therapy dog welfare within sessions. Pending the number of dog-handler teams present for a session, this might involve having a designate whose responsibility is to monitor dog welfare. As a starting point, organizations are responsible for collecting information from handlers attesting to the health of their dog. This might include a veterinarian health certificate, record of vaccines, and fecal test results.

In addition to prioritizing welfare within the organization, the onboarding of new handlers must include both education and training to inform handlers of the importance of therapy dog welfare. This might include training sessions to assist handlers in recognizing and identifying signs of canine stress/distress, establishing protocols within sessions for supporting dogs showing signs of stress, and training handlers around how to best facilitate interactions with clients in ways that reduce stress experienced by dogs (e.g., how to obtain consent).

Handlers

As a starting point and prior to participation in a CAI, handlers are responsible for ensuring their dog is groomed and in optimal physical health and that all documentation regarding their dog's health is up to date and has been submitted per the organization's requirements. Dogs should be exercised and toileted prior to a session to help them settle within their assigned space. To this latter point, dogs who have yet to pass a bowel movement can find settling in a session especially difficult and pre-bowel movement behaviour (or ability to settle and focus on clients) can be markedly different than post-bowel movement behaviour. We've no research to back up this observation – just years of seeing dogs return to a session after a bathroom break easily settle into their role! Another consideration, especially when programs are scheduled during times overlapping with the dog's typically feeding schedule, is that we might see unsettled behaviour in dogs working in programs during their typical feeding time. Adjustments to the dog's feeding schedule could help address this.

Upon arrival to a site, involvement and oversight from the organization's program personnel can vary tremendously and range from program personnel attending and overseeing sessions to organizations not having any on-the-ground presence and rather trusting in handlers to independently represent the organization upholding their values and protocols. Regardless of the level of onsite organizational involvement, handlers bear the bulk of the responsibility in safeguarding and optimizing therapy dog welfare. First, handlers must ensure that the conditions in which their dog is working are comfortable and reflect safety considerations. This might include providing a comfort mat for their dog to lie upon, providing a water bowl, and ensuring their dog is always leashed and under their control.

Second, handlers must provide time for dogs to settle. The experience of a therapy dog, especially those who work in contexts that see multiple dog-handler teams work concurrently in the same shared space, is akin to someone being invited to a party but forbidden from speaking to or interacting with the other guests! There is a lot of self-regulation or ignoring of temptation that is required of therapy dogs. Allowing dogs to settle into the space and becoming familiar with their work station helps them adjust to the demands imposed upon them (see Figure 3.6).

Last, handlers are directly responsible for overseeing the choreography of the interactions that take place between their dog and visiting clients – that is, from the approach of a new client to the interactions that take place during a visit, to the departure of the client. As a starting point, handlers are responsible for *educating* clients around their responsibilities as part of the interaction. This might include how to obtain consent from the dog, how to pet the dog, and the curbing of any undesired behaviours (e.g., overly excitable petting or roughhousing that result in calm dogs becoming agitated). Relatedly, handlers are also responsible for engaging clients throughout the session. This might see handlers share information about their dog (e.g., how the dog was acquired) to information regarding the dog's age, breed, and likes and dislikes. Beyond this informational sharing, handlers may also ask clients questions to find out the motivation for attending a session, whether they have pets at home, and how they're coping (e.g., how a university student is handling the pressures of final exams or how a senior new to a retirement facility is adjusting to their new living situation). As part of this process, handlers are required to demonstrate strong listening skills – not to immediately rush to problem-solving or advice dispensing – but rather to be present with the client as a way of offering support. We'll discuss the skills required of handlers in Chapter 4 when we explore team suitability.

Visiting Clients

Little has been written about the responsibilities of clients who make use of opportunities to interact with therapy dogs. Admittedly, there can be ample variation in the instructions provided to clients with some interactions allowed to unfold organically, whereas others might be more structured (or sequenced). It merits mention too that given the ample variability in the clients supported through CAIs, there too will be variability in clients' abilities to follow directions and adhere to behavioural expectations as laid out by the handler (e.g., a student with exceptional needs as part of a school visit). As noted in the section above, handlers are responsible for guiding the interactions between their therapy dog and members of the public, and visiting clients are responsible for listening to, and following, such instructions. Recall our opening scenario in which a handler prevents an excited high school student from immediately approaching their dog, recognizing that the student's excited state could render the interaction problematic.

In requesting the student take a deep breath to calm themselves, the handler is working to optimize the interaction. Recall that one goal of the therapy dog is to invite the visiting client to match the dog's calm and relaxed state – not the opposite – that an excited student riles an once-calm dog into a excitable frenzy. Thus, visiting clients are to look to handlers for direction, ask permission to approach and interact with the therapy dog, and follow recommendations as explained.

HANDLER'S MENTAL WELL-BEING

Having proffered a definition of therapy dog welfare earlier in this chapter, it is equally important to recognize and define handler welfare. Leveraging the World Health Organization's (2024, para. 1) definition of well-being, we see hander well-being characterized as follows:

"A state of wellbeing in which every individual realizes his or her own potential, can cope with the stress of life, can work productively and fruitfully and is able to make a contribution to his or her community." This definition provides a framework for understanding handler well-being. In it we see themes of resiliency (i.e., able to cope with the stresses of life) and community service or volunteering (i.e., giving of their time to share their dog in sessions supporting visiting clients). In addition to the responsibilities of handlers outlined in the section above, handlers are responsible for arriving to sessions with their mental health optimized. Absent from the literature on therapy dog handlers is a discussion of their mental well-being and the role it plays in guiding the work they do facilitating interactions between their dog and visiting clients. Much of the literature on handlers addresses informational protocols around the management of their dogs and possibly mention of protocols for interacting with clients, but here we see addressing the well-being of handlers as a foundational condition necessary at the outset of the interaction (Table 3.2). Handlers with compromised mental well-being are poorly positioned to oversee the welfare of their dog and to foster well-being in visiting clients – whatever the desired outcome might be (e.g., stress reduction, reduction in loneliness, fostering interpersonal connections, etc.). As an illustration of this point and this might strike readers as obvious however it remains under-addressed and discussed in the literature on training handlers, a handler with elevated stress and anxiety is in no position to facilitate stress and anxiety reduction in visiting clients!

	Recipients	Responsibilities
HANDLER	Themselves	– arrive with optimized well-being
		– remain cognizant of their role, duties, and responsibilities as a handler
		– continued professional education regarding CAIs
	Their dogs	– prepare the dog for participation in the session (e.g., toileting, grooming, etc.)
		– follow arrival and departure procedures as outlined by the institution (e.g., identification for dog, use of designated entrance and exit)
		– ensure a comfort mat and water are made available for dog
		– dog on leash and in control of handler at all times
		– monitor dog welfare throughout the session
	Clients	– educate client on optimal human-dog interactions
		– share information regarding their dog
		– engage the client by asking questions
		– practice active listening/avoid problem-solving
	Organization and broader field	– uphold the vision and mission of the organization
		– serve as an ambassador for the organization

UNDERSTANDING THE INTERPLAY OF EMOTIONS BETWEEN HANDLERS AND DOGS

The notion of *emotional contagion*, the spreading of one individual's emotional state to another individual, warrants discussion as part of the broader discussion of dog-handler team welfare. Although more extensively studied in medical (e.g., Weilenmann et al., 2018) and educational contexts (e.g., Oberle & Schonert-Reichl, 2016), there is but nascent research examining how emotions may be transmitted between humans and animals – here we're concerned with the handler's capacity to convey negative emotional states to the therapy dog working under their charge. In a recent review paper by

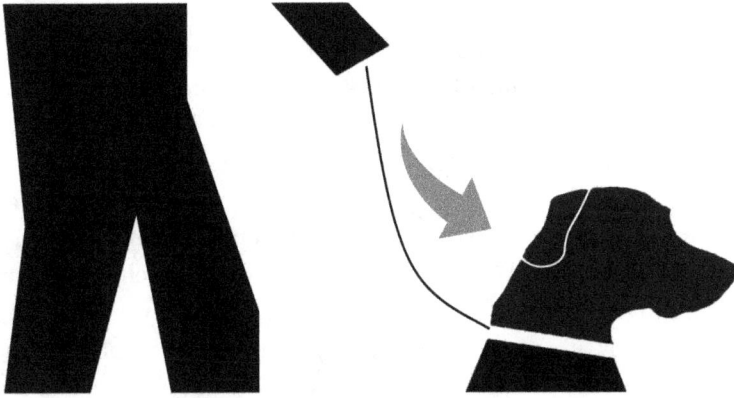

Figure 3.7 Graphic demonstrating that emotions travel from handler to dog

Source: Amanda Lamberti; used with permission

Kong (2022, para. 8), emotional contagion is described as follows: "Emotion contagion research has revealed that exposure to emotional expressions can induce a change in the onlooker's emotional condition. These emotional conditions arise unconsciously and are initiated by cues in the environment that distinctively affect people's mood (Bernsten, 2007)." Hatfield and colleagues (1994) describe the process of passing emotions as *converging emotionally* where one individual adopts, without the intention to do so, the emotional state of another. Thus, a discussion of emotional contagion between a handler and their therapy dog might see negative emotions (e.g., anxiety, worry, stress, agitation, nervousness) transmitted "down-the-leash" to their dog who otherwise was not characterized by these emotions (Figure 3.7).

THE DOWN-THE-LEASH PIPELINE – RECOGNIZING THE POTENTIAL OF EMOTIONAL CONTAGION

Two studies inform our thinking about the transfer of emotions between a handler and their therapy dog. First, in a study of human-to-dog emotional contagion, Katayama and colleagues (2019) examined whether the length of ownership and the strength of the human-animal bond impacted human-to-dog emotional contagion. In a sample of 34 human-dog dyads, these researchers subjected human participants to a public social stressor (i.e., speech preparation, explaining a document, and verbal mental mathematics) and measured electrocardiogram changes in both humans and dogs to identify any subsequent heart rate variability. Findings from a final sample of 14 human-dog dyads (20 pairs were eliminated due to technical difficulties in collecting data) suggest that "…emotional contagion from owner to dog can occur especially in females and the time sharing the same environment is the key factor in inducing the efficacy of emotional contagion." (para. 1). Considering the small sample and methodological challenges in collecting data, we exercise caution in overstating the claims arising from this study. It does however contribute to the body of scientific knowledge attesting to the human-to-dog emotional pipeline that can negatively impact the emotional state of otherwise neutral dogs.

A second study, and one that explicitly examines emotional contagion between handlers and their therapy dogs, is found in research by Silas and colleagues (2019) titled "Therapeutic for all? Observational assessments of therapy canine stress in an on-campus stress-reduction program." In contrast to the study described above, this study had robust participant engagement that saw 40 therapy dog-hander teams and 754 university students complete measures to determine whether participation in an on-campus CAI reduced hander, dog, and student stress and whether there was a link between handler stress and dog stress. Using both human self-reports and observations of therapy dog stress indicators, these authors found that: (1) both handler and student stress significantly decreased from the start to the end of the session; (2) therapy dog stress remained constant from the start to the end of a session; and (3) for handlers who had self-reports of elevated stress, their therapy dogs were characterized by correspondingly higher levels of stress at the end of sessions. Collectively, these findings inform our understanding of the experience therapy dogs have when participating in on-campus CAIs and suggest that handler pre-session stress can negatively impact the therapy dogs working under their charge. This research holds implications for handler training and for the monitoring of dog welfare throughout sessions.

CANINE WELFARE WITHIN RESEARCH

The Role of Ethics in Safeguarding Welfare

Within a research context, researchers are required to prepare and submit applications to research ethics boards for research involving both humans and animals. Broadly, we might consider the Research Ethics Board, certainly within the college or university setting, as a mechanism to safeguard the safety and welfare of therapy dogs. We argue here that the application to conduct research involving therapy dogs is a necessary but insufficient condition for safeguarding therapy dog welfare. In such applications, researchers might be required to report the number of dogs involved in a study, the training and handling procedures of dogs by handlers, the duration of individual sessions and the number of sessions, and whether water and toileting or rest breaks will be provided. Issuing an ethics certificate to conduct research does not guarantee that procedures will be upheld in applied settings and overseeing the actualization of measures to safeguard therapy dog welfare are borne collectively by researchers and their assistants, organization program personnel, and handlers. We recognize that Animal Research Ethics Boards that issue permission for therapy dogs to participate in research protocols may very well be more accustomed to reviewing ethics applications from researchers seeking to do experimental research involving animals in laboratory settings and may be unfamiliar with the nuanced work undertaken by therapy dogs working in CAIs.

The Role of Welfare in Optimizing Intervention Effects

When the welfare of therapy dogs is compromised, they are likely to be less engaged in sessions. This lack of engagement, in turn, can dilute the effects of a CAI. Increasingly, we're seeing researchers report (or perhaps journal reviewers require) how therapy dog welfare was monitored and whether there were any incidents of compromised welfare (e.g., whether any dogs left the study because of elevated stress, etc.). Recall the example provided in Chapter 1 (Figure 1.5) in which we illustrated, from our own research, how researchers might report on the monitoring of therapy dog welfare and any incidents of compromised welfare. This reporting of compromised therapy dog welfare can be especially problematic for researchers as they are agents in the research process with a particularly vested interest in seeing that the intervention is delivered and that data is collected from participants. Halting data collection because a therapy dog is showing signs of distress and sending that team outside for a bathroom break or sending them home can significantly and negatively delay or impact the procedures of a study. It is here we see a call for researchers to put dog-handler team welfare above the need to collect data and to recognize that any data collected from an intervention in which the welfare of the therapy dog is suboptimal is not data reflective of rigorous methodology.

Understanding Factors and Mechanisms Within Interactions

A recent systematic review by Wagner and colleagues (2022) advances the discussion beyond "*Do* animal-assisted interventions work?" to "*How* do animal-assisted interventions work?" This is an important question and one that we address in our discussions of the role of touch in the chapters that follow. As argued by Rodriguez and colleagues (2023, p. 4), "…to build the evidence base of AAIs, it is necessary to isolate the specific effects of the intervention itself, and control for the effects that are not specific to the intervention" (Herzog, 2015). Across studies, there is a collective body of scientific evidence attesting to the efficacy of animal-assisted interventions (AAIs) as a viable way to bolster well-being or reduce ill-being in humans, yet very little is known about the mechanisms at play within interactions between animals and humans. Recall our review of the self-report and biomarker research in Chapter 2 attesting to the efficacy of CAIs on human well-being (Figure 3.8).

Returning to the work of Wagner et al. (2022), to understand the dimensions included in AAIs or excluded and found in control conditions, these authors screened 2,001 AAI studies and analysed 172 studies to identify the specific factors of interventions and compared them to the descriptions of control groups (i.e., the non-specific factors). The idea here was to tease apart the aspects of AAI that researchers introduce as a dimension impacting the efficacy of the AAI. This led Wagner et al. to compile a list reflecting the dimensions or factors of AAIs that have been experimentally manipulated and a list of the dimensions or non-specific factors incorporated into control conditions (see Table 3.3).

Two salient observations emerge from this list that inform the advancement of AAI research. First, researchers, to date, have tested relatively few dimensions of AAIs (see Specific Factors column in Table 3.3). Additional research elucidating the mechanisms undergirding AAIs is warranted to respond to the question "How do AAIs work?" This is echoed by the author Angela Fournier (2019, vii) who posited: "There

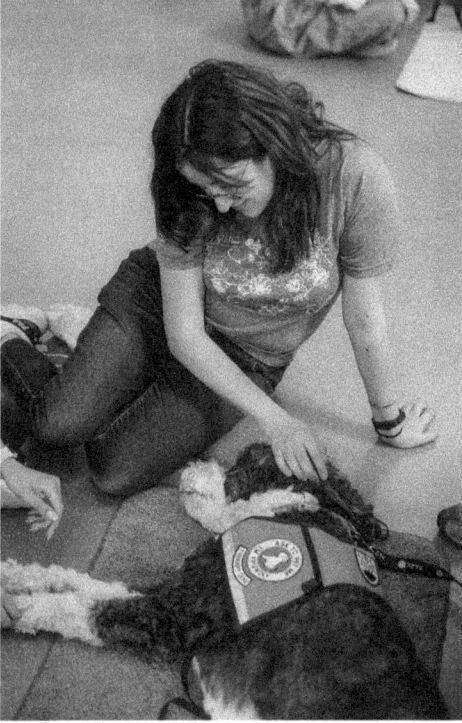

Figure 3.8 An undergraduate student sits with therapy dog Daisy, a Sheepadoodle, and gently touches her ears

Source. Freya L. L. Green Photography; used with permission

is very little study of just how humans and animals interact and which interactions or features of the animal are therapeutic." Second, and as reflected by the varied factors introduced in the control conditions of the studies examined (see Non-Specific Factors column in Table 3.3), there is ample variability in how researchers have crafted control conditions – conditions that allow them to approximate the intervention condition but without the key aspect of interacting with an animal. Thus, we see approximations of sorts where study participants in control conditions might interact with a (non-live) proxy animal (i.e., a stuffed or robotic animal) or participate in reflective or mindfulness exercises.

It merits mention that when conducting CAI research involving randomized controlled trials where study participants are assigned to intervention (with a therapy dog) or control (no therapy dog)

Table 3.3 Factors Found Within AAIs

Specific Factors Inherent in AAIs	Non-specific Factors Inherent in AAIs
Animal	Therapeutic dimensions
Interactions taking place within sessions	Opportunity for social interactions/engagement
Animal's movement	Extent of physical activity/movement
Extent of physical contact between client and animal	Activity, distraction, or distortion
Care of animal/animal husbandry	Education or training
Other factors (e.g., use of specialized equipment, frequency of interactions)	Plush or toy animal
	The participating animal
	Contextual environment
	Interacting with a proxy animal (e.g., riding a mechanical horse)
	Movement or rhythm
	Relaxations
	Watching/observing an animal
	Novelty
	Other (e.g., dimensions of the control condition not fitting any of the above categories)

Source: Adapted from Wagner et al. (2022)

conditions, participants in the control condition can be dismayed to learn they were not selected or provided the opportunity to interact with a therapy dog. Using a wait-list control group where participants have an opportunity at the end of the study to interact with therapy dogs is one step to try and alleviate this dismay. In recent research by Green and Binfet (2023), 280 undergraduate students (77% women, Mage = 20.2 years, 62% white) were assigned to direct touch, close proximity to a therapy dog but no touch, or no dog conditions. In open-ended prompts, participants were quick to share their negative views at not being assigned to their preferred condition with 30% of participants in the close proximity but no touch condition offering negative comments, compared to 13% of participants in the no-dog/handler-only condition, followed by 4% of participants in the touch condition offering negative views on their experience in the study (see Green & Binfet, 2023, for full study results here). In our last chapter (Chapter 8), we will explore the areas for future research that address these and other challenges raised in CAI and AAI research.

In addition to the above observations informing future research arising from Wagner et al.,'s (2022) systematic review, so too are there ramifications for animal welfare inherent in their findings. Granted we are not so bothered by the variability in the non-specific dimensions of the control groups used by AAI researchers (as there is no animal present or participating in these conditions), however the introduction of specific factors or mechanisms into AAIs can create conditions in which therapy animals are subject to participating in studies with novel introductions – aspects of studies not previously empirically tested. Revisiting Wagner et al.'s specific factor list, we see researchers have introduced movement, equipment, and directed the nature of interactions to include, for example, touch. The introduction of modifications or manipulations to the independent variable (i.e., the AAI itself) must be done with research ethics' approval, care, and consideration for the experience and welfare of the dog-handler teams, and introduced with strong welfare oversight.

MEASURING PARTICIPANTS' ENGAGEMENT IN SESSIONS

Much of our discussion throughout this chapter has focussed on dog and handler welfare and how welfare can compromise or optimize the team's participation in CAIs. We have argued above that both therapy dogs and handlers are agents in the CAI who play key roles in helping ensure that the CAI was delivered as intended. This reflects *implementation fidelity* – the extent to which the independent variable was delivered as outlined in the methodological design of the study. Researchers should be concerned with implementation fidelity and report steps taken to ensure that the CAI was actualized as intended. Steps to enhance implementation fidelity might include the careful screening and training of dog-handler teams, providing handlers a bank of questions to use to foster interactions with study participants, and predetermining the duration of the session to determine participants' exposure to the independent variable – the CAI.

Related to the above discussion yet often overlooked in CAI research is any measurement of participants' engagement in the CAI. That is, to what extent and how did participants participate in the intervention? Were they passive? Were they playful and interactive with the dogs? Did they engage with handlers by responding to questions and engage in dialogue? Efforts have been made to measure the extent to which participants engaged with dogs within the CAI (see Figure 3.9). Using

---

Engagement Questionnaire

Help us understand your interaction with the therapy dog. For this session, how engaged were you? Engagement is demonstrated through eye contact, physically touching, and proximity to the therapy dog.

Rate each of these engagement dimensions for your session today:

1. I made **eye contact** with the therapy dog:

1	2	3	4	5
Not Often				Very Often

2. My **physical proximity** to the dog was:

1	2	3	4	5
Not Close				Very Close

3. I **physically touched** (petted) the therapy dog:

1	2	3	4	5
Not Often				Very Often

THANK YOU FOR COMPLETING THIS SURVEY. NEXT, YOU ARE ASKED TO RETURN YOUR BOOKLET TO A MEMBER OF THE RESEARCH TEAM. THANK YOU AGAIN FOR YOUR CONTRIBUTION TO ADVANCING CANADIAN SCIENCE AROUND CANINE-ASSISTED INTERVENTIONS.

Figure 3.9 Open-ended survey prompts to measure participant engagement within a session

rating scales to measure eye contact, the proximity to the dog, and the extent to which participants engaged in touch by petting or caressing the therapy dog, can collectively provide an estimate of the extent to which participants were engaged in the intervention. Likewise, researchers might ask study participants about their engagement with handlers to get a comprehensive sense of how participants interacted with the dog-handler team.

CONCLUSION

The aim of this chapter was to proffer a definition of therapy dog welfare and examine the roles of various agents involved in the organization and delivery of CAIs in safeguarding welfare. In doing so, we raised issues germane to optimizing both dog and handler welfare and examined concepts such as emotional contagion between handlers and their dogs, how signs of canine stress might be the dog coping with within-session stress, and how less than optimal dog welfare can dilute the quality of the intervention in research studies. In Chapter 4 that follows, we examine dog-handler team suitability and examine the dispositions and behaviours that contribute to handlers and therapy dogs excelling within CAIs.

REFERENCES

Berntsen, D. (2007). Involuntary autobiographical memories: Speculations, findings and an attempt to integrate them. In J. H. Mace (Ed.), *Involuntary memory* (pp. 20–50). https://doi.org/10.1002/9780470774069

Chandler, C. (2012). *Animal assisted therapy in counseling*. Routledge. https://doi.org/10.4324/9780203832103

Clark, S. D., Smidt, J. M., & Bauer, B. A. (2020). Therapy dogs' and handlers' behavior and salivary cortisol during initial visits in a complex medical institution: A pilot study. *Frontiers in Veterinary Science, 7*, 564201. https://www.frontiersin.org/journals/veterinary-science/articles/10.3389/fvets.2020.564201/full

Eaton-Stull, Y. M., Jaffe, B., Scott, K., & Shiller, M. (2023). Animal-assisted crisis response: Characteristics of canine handlers and their canine partners. *Human-Animal Interactions, 11*(1). https://doi.org/10.1079/hai.2023.0033

Fournier, A. K. (2019). *Animal-assisted intervention: Thinking empirically*. Cham, Switzerland: Palgrave MacMillian.

Green, F. L. L., & Binfet, J. T. (2023). Beyond cuddling canines: Exploring students' perceptions of the importance of touch in an on-campus canine-assisted intervention. *Emerging Adulthood, 11*(5), 1238–1254. https://doi.org/10.1177/2167696 8231188754

Hatfield, E., Cacioppo, J. T., & Rapson, R. L. (1994). Emotional contagion. *Review of Personality and Social Psychology*, 14, 151–177.

Herzog, H. (2015). The research challenge: Threats to the validity of animal-assisted therapy studies and suggestions for improvements. In Fine, A. H. (Ed.), *Handbook of animal-assisted therapy: Foundations and guidelines for animal-assisted interventions 4th ed.* (pp. 402–407). Academic Press.

Hetts, S., Clark, J. D., Arnold, C. E., & Mateo, J. M. (1992). Influence of housing conditions on beagle behaviour. *Applied Animal Behavior Science*, 34, 137–155.

Katayama, M., Kubo, T., Yamakawa, T., Fujiwara, K., Nomoto, K., . . . Kikusui, T. (2019). Emotional contagion from humans to dogs is facilitated by duration of ownership. *Frontiers in Psychology*, 10, 1678. https://doi.org/10.3389/fpsyg.2019.01678

Kong, Y. (2022). Are emotions contagious? A conceptual review of studies in language education. *Frontiers in Psychology*, 13, 1048105. https://doi.org/10.3389/fpsyg.2022.1048105

Lackey, R., & Haberstock, G. (2019). Animal-assisted crisis response: Offering opportunity for human resiliency during and after traumatic incidents. In P. Tedeschi & M. A. Jenkins (Eds.), *Transforming trauma: Resilience and healing through our connections with animals* Purdue University Press. https://www.jstor.org/stable/j.ctv2x00vgg.16

Ng, Z., Albright, J., Fine, A. H., & Peralta, J. (2015). Our ethical and moral responsibility: Ensuring the welfare of therapy animals. In A. Fine (Ed.), *Handbook on animal-assisted therapy* (4th ed., (pp. 357–376). Elsevier.

Novak, M. A., & Drewsen, K. H. (1989). Enriching the lives of captive primates: Issues and problems. In E. F. Segal (Ed.), *Housing, care, and psychological wellbeing of captive and laboratory primates* (pp. 161–185). Noyes.

Oberle, E., & Schonert-Reichl, K. A. (2016). Stress contagion in the classroom? The link between classroom teacher burnout and morning cortisol in elementary school students. *Social Science & Medicine*, 159, 30–37. https://doi.org/10.1016/j.socscimed.2016.04.031

Pastore, C., Pirrone, F., Balzarotti, F., Faustini, M., Pierantoni, L., & Albertini, M. (2011). Evaluation of physiological and behavioral stress-dependent parameters in agility dogs. *Journal of Veterinary Behavior*, 6, 188–194. https://doi.org/10.1016/j.jveb.2011.01.001

Rodriguez, K. E., Green, F. L. L., Binfet, J. T., Townsend, L., & Gee, N. (2023). Complexities and considerations in conducting animal-assisted intervention research: A discussion of randomized controlled trials. *Human–Animal Interactions*. https://doi.org/10.1079/hai.2023.0004

Shiverdecker, M. D., Schiml, P. A., & Hennessy, M. B. (2013). Human interaction moderates plasma cortisol and behavioral responses of dogs to shelter housing. *Physiology & Behavior*, 109, 75–79. https://doi.org/10.1016/j.physbeh.2012.12.002

Silas, H. J., Binfet, J. T., & Ford, A. (2019). Therapeutic for all? Observational assessments of therapy canine stress in an on-campus stress reduction program. *Journal of Veterinary Behavior: Clinical Applications and Research*, 32, 6–13. https://doi.org/10.1016/j.jveb.2019.03.009

Stewart, L. A., Bruneau, L., & Elliot, A. (2016). The role of animal-assisted interventions in addressing trauma-informed care. Available at: https://www.counseling.org/knowledge-center/vistas/by-subject2/vistas-aniaml-assisted/docs/default-source/vistas/article_4690fd25f16116603abcacff0000bee5e7.

Wagner, C., Grob, C., & Hediger, K. (2022). Specific and non-specific factors of animal-assisted interventions considered in research: A systematic review. *Frontiers in Psychology*, 13, 931347. https://doi.org/10.3389/fpsyg.2022.931347

Weilenmann, S., Schnyder, U., Parkinson, B., Corda, C., von Känel, R., & Pfaltz, M. C. (2018). Emotion transfer, emotion regulation, and empathy-related processes in physician-patient interactions and their association with physician well-being: A theoretical model. *Frontiers in Psychiatry*, 9, 389. https://doi.org/10.3389/fpsyt.2018.00389

World Health Organization (2024). https://www.paho.org/en/topics/mental-health#:~:text=The%20World%20Health%20Organization%20(WHO,to%20his%20or%20her%20community%E2%80%9D.

Four

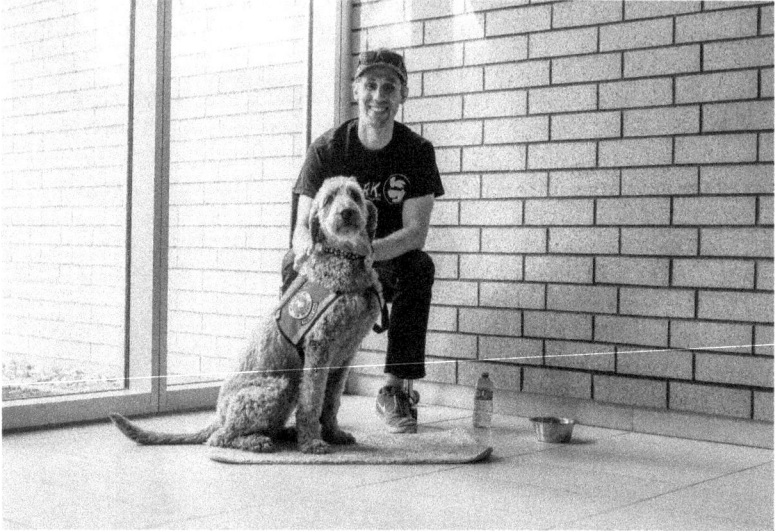

Figure 4.1 Handler Adam settles his therapy dog Ginny at their station as they prepare to meet visiting clients. For appropriate identification at the facility, Adam is wearing the organization's team shirt and Ginny is wearing her red therapy dog vest

Source: F. L. L. Green Photography; used with permission

DOI: 10.4324/9781032639284-4

SCENARIO

Would You Like Fries with Your Interaction?

Carrying a takeout container of French fries, a young man wearing a large backpack approaches Candice and her therapy dog, a volunteer dog-handler team working in a busy airport terminal to support stressed travellers. With a mouthful of food, the young man asks, "Hey, can your dog have a French fry? My dog loves fries!" Without waiting for an answer, the young man drops French fries on the floor. Although well behaved and having previously practiced the "leave it" command, Candice's dog Bella grabs several fries before Candice has time to direct her otherwise. In frustration, Candice says, "Are you kidding me?" tugs on Bella's leash and walks away from the young traveller. In debriefing her volunteer time with the program director later that week, Candice shared "I'll admit I could have handled that better. I missed an opportunity to educate the guy on how to interact. I knew to expect the unexpected when volunteering at the airport but I didn't think I'd be fighting off French fries! Things like this should be included in your handler orientation training."

QUESTIONS FOR DISCUSSION AND REFLECTION

1. Should therapy dogs work in busy public settings where factors undermining welfare can be unpredictable and challenging to control?

2. How might the context in which therapy dogs work undermine welfare?

3. What are the behavioural expectations for the public when interacting with therapy dogs?

4. What are the behavioural expectations for dogs and food in public spaces?

5. How can handlers proactively manage their surroundings while remaining open, inviting, and engaging with potential visitors?

In Figure 4.1, we see a handler identified with a program shirt, their dog wearing an identification vest, the dog secured by a leash, a comfort mat provided, as well as water for both the dog and the handler. Also, in this photo, we note that the dog-handler team is positioned in a way that prevents clients from surprising them from behind, thus optimizing the dog's sense of security within this working environment. The aim of this chapter is to examine and elucidate the characteristics, dispositions, skills, and behaviours of therapy dogs and handlers that are required of teams to successfully support clients in a range of settings. Introduced earlier, this chapter begins with an applied scenario in which a handler encounters the unexpected when volunteering in an airport, and over the course of this chapter, we'll refer to the challenge in this scenario as we identify the characteristics of dog-handler teams and their suitability for work in delivering canine-assisted interventions (CAIs).

ACCESSING DOG-HANDLER TEAMS

There appear to be two distinct pathways through which we see therapy dogs accessed by the public. First, dog-handler teams may be outsourced from a therapy dog organization or agency for participation in various programming to support clients at different locations (e.g., a team of dog handlers is booked for a middle-school visit to support the school's Mental Health Week); and second, individuals might take it upon themselves to develop protocols to assess their own dog-handler teams (i.e., a "within-house" approach). The advantages and limitations of each approach are discussed next.

Outsourcing Dog-Handler Teams

There are several advantages to outsourcing dog-handler teams and these include: (1) all vetting of dogs and their handlers has been conducted; (2) the organization oversees the training of handlers for participation in CAIs, and the dogs and handlers are likely to be experienced, having participated in other programs. They thus bring a certain level of expertise when booked for a session and are familiar with how to set up stations and how to engage clients; and (3) any issues of liability are borne by the organization outsourcing the teams, thus reducing the burden on those who book the visit.

We must consider too the disadvantages of outsourcing dog-handler teams. This can include: (1) information regarding the training and expertise of the organizational personnel can be difficult to discern (i.e., do personnel have formal training and experience in the assessment of dog-hander teams?); (2) a lack of transparency in how dogs and handlers are vetted (e.g., Is a criminal record check required annually from handlers? Have all dogs been assessed to work with a range of clients including children?); (3) the quality of training provided to handlers may vary (or whether training has even been provided); and (4) there may be constraints around the number of dog-handler teams available, the availability of teams, and the locations served by teams.

In-House Organization Dog-Handler Team Assessments

At the outset, it's important to recognize that not all geographic areas are served by therapy dog associations, organizations, or agencies, and conducting in-house assessments may be the only option to generate access to therapy dog-handler teams. It merits noting that this might not always be the case as it could be that an agency seeking to access therapy dogs wants to customize their approach to vetting dog-handler teams and feels this oversight is essential to the success of the program. In this regard, the assessment of teams may be conducted knowing the context where teams will work and knowing the nature of the client to be served. Examples of this might include dog-handler teams working in an inner-city, after-school program where nuanced handler knowledge and interactions are required to support children or dog-handler teams working in a busy police detachment to support officer stress reduction where advanced security screenings of the handlers and additional training of the teams are needed to work in this challenging context (see Binfet et al., 2020; Green & Binfet, 2021). Readers are directed to information provided by Pet Partners (2022) titled "Starting a Program at Your Facility" that outlines considerations such as creating buy-in and consulting varied agents or groups in the planning process.

The advantages of conducting in-house credentialling are that the dog-handler teams can be assessed and evaluated knowing the clients they'll support. It could be that dog-handler teams work uniquely in one setting in support of one type of client (e.g., therapy dogs supporting lonely seniors in a large residential care facility). In this regard, the credentialling of the team can be nuanced, and the training and education provided can be geared to meeting the needs of this particular group (e.g., familiarizing dogs with mobility aids frequently used by seniors). Another advantage of in-house credentialling is that dog-handler teams can reach "hard to reach clients" that would otherwise not be served by any outsourced dog-handler teams. Such might be the case in geographically remote or rural settings where a rich pool of credentialled dog-handler teams is unavailable. Related to having dog-handler teams assessed with specific clients in mind, so too can modifications be made for dog-handler teams with exceptional or special needs. Such might be the case for dogs or handlers with mobility issues or hearing impairments. Considering the exceptional needs of dogs and handlers during team assessments can help diversify the profiles of both the therapy dogs and handlers we see volunteering in CAIs.

Just as we saw disadvantages in *outsourcing* dog-handler teams, so too can there be disadvantages or limitations with the *in-house* approach to certifying therapy dogs and their handlers. First, the credentials, education, background, or formal training of the individuals within the organization who are responsible for assessing and evaluating dog-handler teams can vary tremendously and can potentially compromise the quality and sophistication of the credentialling process. The field of human-animal interactions (HAIs) is known to be interdisciplinary, and it's not uncommon to see researchers from a variety of fields interested in interventions and programs involving therapy dogs (e.g., psychology, education, social work, nursing, anthrozoology, veterinary medicine).

Equally in applied programming, we see the background of individuals vary and range from those who are self-taught to having pursued graduate studies with a focus on animal behaviour. In short, there is ample variability in the range of qualifications of individuals who undertake the assessment and evaluation of therapy dog-handler teams, and, resultingly, we see wide variability in the competencies and skills of these individuals and their ability to create a process to discern dog-handler teams who are optimally suited to undertake work in support of clients in varied contexts. Added to this, *in-house* operations may also be understaffed with personnel fulfilling multiple roles concurrently. For example, the same individual may be responsible for credentialling teams, updating all of the teams' health profiles and overseeing record keeping, liaising with the public, monitoring dog welfare, and providing ongoing professional development to handlers – or doing little of this. The scope of the work required to successfully oversee a therapy dog organization, even *in-house*, can be daunting and requires an understanding of dog behaviour, therapy dog skills, and knowledge of the target clients to be supported including the context they're in.

When Therapy Dogs Are Unavailable

When neither of the two above options – *outsourcing* therapy dog-handler teams from an established agency or credentialling dog-handler teams through *in-house* assessment, we can see informal opportunities emerge that strive to meet the demand to interact with dogs. One example of this is found in events described as "Bring your dog to work." Oftentimes held on university or college campuses, these events encourage employees to bring their dog to work "providing the dog is friendly" and provide time for employees to gather to share their dog with fellow co-workers or the broader public. A second example is found in educators who, recognizing the benefits of having a dog in school on the school climate, interpersonal interactions, and student behaviour, bring their dog to their school on a regular basis. There are other iterations of this informal incorporation of companion dogs into public spaces; however, these two illustrations are, by far, the most common informal examples we see of dogs serving as *pseudo-therapy dogs*.

There are many dangers and risks arising from this informal intro duction of companion dogs into public spaces. First, without any formal assessment of the dog's temperament, competencies, and skills or the vetting of the owner's ability to manage their dog, there is a risk of injury to members of the public. Dogs who are friendly with adults can respond differently to, and be less accepting of, children. Dogs can have reactions to people's clothing, mobility devices, gender, and skin tone, and if a dog is interacting with the public, as is the case with companion dogs brought to campus for a "pet day," serious consequences can result. Second, oftentimes these events bring together many dogs at once and inter-dog aggression poses a threat as dogs may not enjoy interacting with, and sharing space with, one or several other dogs (again who are managed with variability by their owners). Third, when employees bring their companion dogs to work, whether it be a college campus or a high school, these employees are still required to perform their work duties and functions. That is, the workday and all its corresponding tasks must still be performed and the dog is required to tag along, the whole day long, as these tasks are completed. In this regard, the employee has a bifurcated responsibility – perform work duties whilst managing their dog. Fourth, in addition to the long hours, there may be environmental hazards that compromise the welfare of companion dogs brought into public spaces. These might include but are not limited to elevated temperatures, inconsistent access to water, dropped food/medication, unfamiliar noises, machinery, or technology, and over-enthusiastic interactions by well-meaning co-workers or students. Collectively, the positioning of companion dogs as pseudo-therapy dogs raises all kinds of risks – to employees, to the public, and especially with respect to compromising dog welfare.

THERAPY DOGS – A UNIQUE CLASSIFICATION OF WORKING DOGS

As discussed briefly in Chapter 2, there are many different types of helping or working dogs (e.g., dogs for the hearing impaired, guide dogs for the visually impaired, psychiatric service dogs, emotional support dogs, etc.), and therapy dogs are unique in that they are one of the few dogs that provide service to multiple client recipients, often at the same time. Whereas a service dog is likely to support but one individual to optimize their ability to live independently, a therapy dog may provide support to a wide array of individuals and multiple individuals at the same time. In this regard, the skills required of a therapy dog to adapt to varied settings and to a variety of clients render the work they do especially challenging (see Figure 4.2). Next, we examine the dispositions and skills required of both handlers and their therapy dogs for participation in CAIs (Figure 4.3).

DISPOSITIONS AND SKILLS OF HANDLERS

In an extant review of the HAI and animal-assisted intervention (AAI) literature, there is a paucity of research and information on the dispositions and skills required of handlers within the context of CAIs. Just what makes a strong and competent handler? In the last chapter (Chapter 3), we explored some of the responsibilities of handlers as they oversee interactions with the public and next, and we explore and examine more deeply the qualities of handlers that optimize their ability to facilitate interactions between their therapy dog and clients.

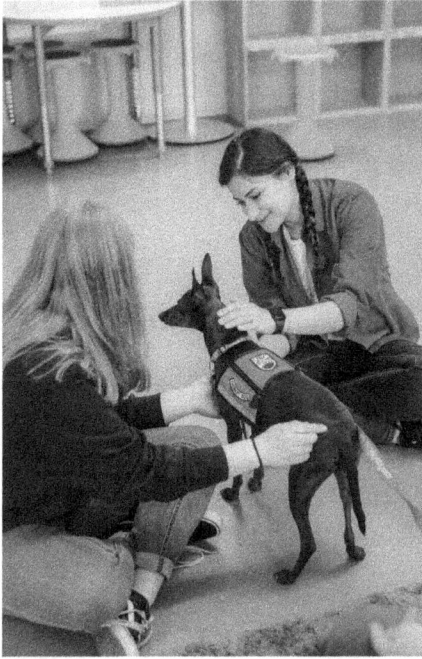

Figure 4.2 A graduate student shares a tender moment with an undergraduate student and therapy dog Canele, a rescued Italian Greyhound

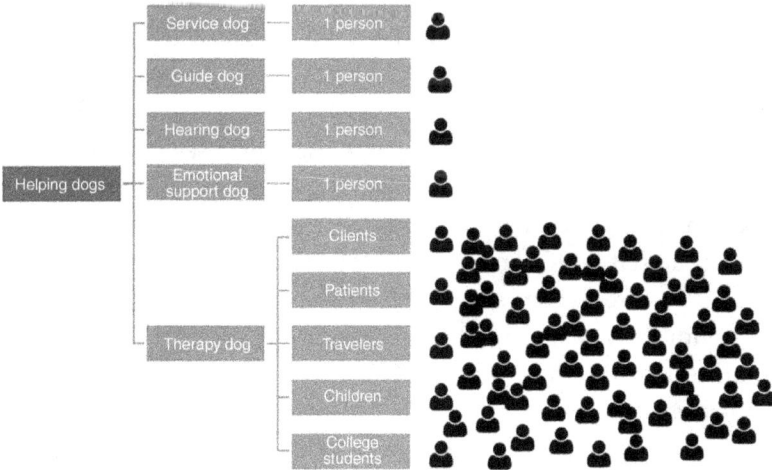

Figure 4.3 Illustration of the high variety and number of clients supported by therapy dogs in comparison with other helping dogs

Source: Binfet & Hartwig, 2020; used with permission

Dispositions

A disposition is described as "the natural qualities of a person's character" and is synonymous with a person's temperament (Oxford Learner's Dictionaries, 2024). Within the context of volunteer work as a therapy dog handler, the handler should have dispositions that align with their varied roles and with the outcomes they're seeking to support in the clients with whom they interact. As an illustration of this latter point and one highlighted in Chapter 3, a handler who themselves arrives to a session with elevated stress is poorly positioned to reduce the stress of college students attending a drop-in CAI and may even increase the stress of their own therapy dog. Considering the varied roles that handlers fulfill, we see the following subcategories.

Ambassador for the Therapy Dog Organization

The handler serves as an ambassador for the broader therapy dog organization and the more immediate program for which they volunteer. Recall the French fry incident faced by Candice and her dog Bella working in a busy airport to support stressed travellers depicted in our opening scenario. Here we saw a handler and her dog working independently in a busy public context on behalf of an organization that facilitates access to dog-handler teams for another organization (i.e., the airport). In this role and as part of the interactions she'd have with the public, Candice would field questions about the therapy dog program, and members of the public would likely ask what it takes to become a volunteer. Candice should be aware of the mission or vision of the organization for which she volunteers and be able to share information with members of the public seeking additional information about what they do and the services they offer. As we live in a technology-driven world where photographs are routinely taken, Candice herself should be mindful that she and her dog abide by identification or dress codes as stipulated by her organization (e.g., have a shirt with the organization logo, dog wearing a vest, etc.). Handlers volunteering with their dog in public settings might also facilitate the recruitment of future handlers for the organization. That is, handlers may encourage members of the public to apply to the organization to bolster volunteer numbers.

In addition to serving as an ambassador for the therapy dog organization for which they volunteer, handlers bear the brunt of responsibility with respect to safeguarding, optimizing, and ensuring their dog's physical safety and emotional welfare. Depending on the size and sophistication of the program for which they volunteer, there may be program personnel assigned to monitor canine welfare. We suspect this is the exception rather than the rule; handlers are largely left to safeguard their dog's welfare within sessions as they often find themselves working independently and not under the direct supervision or guidance of program personnel. Revisiting the definition of therapy dog welfare introduced in Chapter 3 helps elucidate the handler's responsibilities around dog welfare.

> Therapy dog welfare within a CAI is a state of well-being monitored and facilitated by a handler that sees the dog consent to an interaction with a human, demonstrates behaviours reflecting that the interaction is welcomed (e.g., prompting the human for additional petting, leaning into client, etc.), demonstrates behaviour free of agitation or distress (i.e., excessive panting, shaking, whale eye, etc.), and where the dog has the freedom to retreat from the interaction of their own freewill (i.e., not crowded and with a pathway to retreat) without negative consequences (i.e., redirection or correction from handler).

Embedded within this definition, we see the following responsibilities of handlers vis-à-vis their dog's welfare.

- The constant monitoring of their dog's behaviour within a session for signs of stress
- Facilitating interactions with the public in ways that respect the dog's welfare (i.e., establishing consent, watching for signs the dog welcomes additional interaction, etc.)
- Ensuring their dog does not experience crowding and is always able to retreat from an interaction

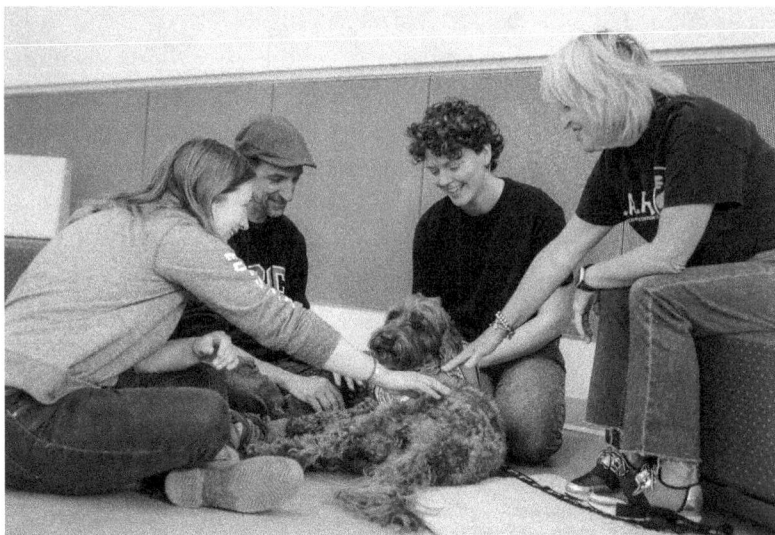

Figure 4.4 Handler Deb facilitates interactions between her therapy dog, Cali, and three young adults. Cali relaxes on a client's lap as two others gently pet her

Source: Freya L. L. Green Photography; used with permission

- Monitoring the number of interactions their dog is asked to do (i.e., the number of new clients within a session) and the duration of their working time
- Honouring their dog's decision to not continue working (e.g., possibly offering a break or ending a session entirely)

Source of Support for Visiting Clients

In addition to serving as an ambassador for the therapy dog organization and safeguarding their dog's physical and emotional welfare within a session, handlers serve as a source of support to the clients with whom they interact. Depending on the type of program in which they volunteer, handlers can support clients characterized by an array of emotional states (i.e., from low to high affect) within a variety of different contexts. For example, on college campuses where students' rates of loneliness are known to be elevated, an interaction between a student and a handler may be the only positive and meaningful interaction a student has the entire week.

Comparably, within the context of a CAI within a residential care facility that sees seniors interact with dog-handler teams, a visit with a handler might be the only visit from a non-staff member the resident experiences that week. In this regard, the handler must have strong perspective-taking skills and be cognizant of the significance of the interaction in the eyes of the client. Especially for clients who do not have regular access to dogs, an interaction with a therapy dog can be especially moving and meaningful. It can recall memories for a student of a family dog back home with one's parents or for a senior of a cherished family pet hoping for dropped tidbits from beneath the kitchen table.

It's important to note too that, for some clients, it will become apparent to the handler that additional support, well beyond the capabilities, mission, and scope of the CAI, is required (e.g., a university student discloses ideas of self-harm). The handler is thus responsible for notifying program personnel that additional support may be warranted so that the client can be directed to additional services (i.e., it is not the role of the handler to deliver these services but rather to act as a conduit for the client to access additional support).

SKILLS

There are a variety of skills required by handlers, and they fall neatly into the subcategories of *Dog Handling Skills* and *Intra- and Interpersonal Skills*. Each is discussed next.

Dog Handling Skills

A skilled handler is one who can manage their dog in public whilst allowing their dog sufficient freedom to engage clients. Next, we'll examine the dog handling skills required by handlers to optimize interactions.

A Proactive Approach

A proactive versus reactive outlook or approach to managing their dog when in public can help avoid conflict and maintain a healthy handler-dog bond. From the parking lot to the session site, the handler must be aware of their surroundings and guide their dog while avoiding potential hazards. As public spaces are known to contain hazards (e.g., glass from a broken bottle, food trash, etc.), the handler must be on the lookout as they make their way to sessions. Some programs see multiple dog-handler teams work concurrently, and handlers must lead their dog to sessions, knowing they may cross paths with other dogs.

Revisiting Candice and her dog Bella in the opening scenario, had Candice seen the young traveller approaching her carrying food, she might have been able to establish parameters to support a successful interaction (e.g., "We'll wait over here until you finish your fries."). We're not naïve to think anticipating all possible hazards is possible but maintain the stance that being proactive *en route* to and within sessions helps reduce the handler expending energy in reactively addressing hazards or resolving conflicts.

A handler who employs a proactive approach might anticipate their dog needing a break BEFORE the dog signals that it needs a break. In this regard, the handler would be mindful of how long the dog has been working, how busy the context is and the tally of clients interacted with, and the overall climate or energy in the room. Collectively, these factors and others can inform the handler that a pre-emptive break is needed to avoid compromising the dog's welfare. Again, a proactive approach to handling doesn't wait for the dog to signal to the handler that they're at the tipping point. Rather, the tipping point (the point where the dog clearly indicates they are not enjoying the CAI and want a break or to leave) is avoided entirely. Here, the handler knowing their dog well, having a secure attachment with their dog, and being informed of signs or indicators of stress/distress, all inform the handler's awareness to initiate a proactive step to protect their dog's welfare.

Fostering Secure Handler-Dog Attachment

Building on our discussion of dog-handler attachment in Chapter 2 and our experience of assessing and evaluating dog-handler teams, one red flag that compromises a team's ability to interact with clients and support their well-being is when there is an insecure attachment characterizing the handler-dog bond. A dog who is uniquely handler-focussed will show little interest in visiting clients and may even perceive these outsiders as a threat to their connection to the handler. In contrast, when a secure human-dog attachment is evident, the dog sees the handler as a secure anchor or source of safety. This, in turn, affords the dog the confidence to explore within the immediate environment, including seeking connections with visiting clients. In Chapter 7, we'll explore and illustrate how a team might be assessed for their handler-dog attachment.

Allowing Therapy Dogs to Work Intuitively

Regarding handlers managing or directing their dogs, it remains important for handlers to not over-control their dogs and allow them to work intuitively. That is, handlers must provide a certain sense of freedom for dogs to act on their intuition. An overmanaged dog has little opportunity to exercise such intuition. We've not seen published research on the intuition of therapy dogs to identify or respond to clients who "need them most" – the idea that therapy dogs are able to connect and support the clients who perhaps arrive with fragile emotions. We'll raise this topic again in our last chapter (Chapter 8) under Future Directions as research is needed to understand intuition in therapy dogs.

As an illustration of this intuition at work, consider the experience of a faculty member on a busy campus who volunteers in an on-campus CAI and who, against campus policy, had their well-behaved therapy dog with them as they headed from one meeting to the next, the dog known for its consistent off-leash heal. Entering the elevator, the faculty member noticed their dog had strayed and, upon glancing out into the corridor, saw a tall lanky first-year Engineering student hunched over their dog, tears streaming down his cheeks and onto the dog who'd stopped to greet him. As the faculty member approached, the student shared, "He knew I needed him. I just failed another midterm and am having a hard time. A real hard time." Anecdotal in nature for sure, but there's something about the intuitive sense or nature of therapy dogs that requires additional discussion and exploration. The takeaway here is that, for therapy dogs to connect to clients, they shouldn't be overmanaged or controlled by handlers – they must have the freedom to do what they do best – connect with clients. Therapy dogs must be under the control of their handlers, but some room within interactions to allow dogs to work intuitively should be considered.

The field of Social and Emotional Learning (SEL) is a discipline that studies and explicates the intra- (i.e., within the individual) and inter- (i.e., between individuals) processes through which people learn to navigate, and cope with, varied social and emotional dimensions of life (see Appendix 4.1). The Collaborative for Academic and Social and Emotional Learning (CASEL; CASEL.org), a repository of all things SEL, offers a definition of SEL that informs the skills required by handlers.

> SEL is the process through which all young people and adults acquire and apply the knowledge, skills, and attitudes to develop health identities, manage emotions and achieve personal and collective goals, feel and show empathy for others, establish and maintain positive supportive relationships, and make responsible and caring decisions (CASEL.org).

Initially proffered as a framework to understand and promote the development of children and adolescents in school, the CASEL model of social and emotional competencies has been reconfigured to include families and communities. It is this latter positioning of the SEL competencies that we leverage as we explore the skills required of handlers in their role in CAIs. Within the definition above, we see both intra- and interpersonal social and emotional skills and competencies (see Table 4.1). We assert that the stronger the handler's social and emotional competencies, the better able they are to manage themselves, manage their dog, welcome and support clients within sessions, and profit from their volunteer experience. Having explored the dispositions and skills of handlers, next, we turn our attention to a discussion of the dispositions and skills required of therapy dogs.

DISPOSITIONS AND BEHAVIOURS OF THERAPY DOGS

It's important to keep in mind that the extent to which therapy dogs possess the dispositions and behaviours characterizing strong and competent therapy dogs, the better positioned they'll be to withstand the stressors that arise in working in a public setting in support

Table 4.1 An Illustration of Social and Emotional Core Competencies Informing the Handler Role

Intrapersonal Skills	Description	Application to Handlers
Self-Awareness	– Identifying emotions – Accurate – self-perception – Recognizing strengths – Self-confidence – Self-efficacy	Handlers must have the confidence to manage their dog in public, meet and introduce their dog to the public, and engage the public via interactions with their therapy dog.
Self-Management	– Impulse control – Stress management – Self-discipline – Self-motivation – Goal setting – Organizational skills	Handlers must practice self-regulation as they avoid dispensing advice to clients (i.e., problem-solving) and refer clients to outside available resources to address their needs beyond the support offered in a CAI. Handlers must arrive to sessions with optimal well-being recognizing the role that emotional contagion can play in impacting both dogs and visiting clients.
Responsible Decision-Making	– Identifying problems – Analyzing situations – Solving problems – Evaluating – Reflecting – Ethical responsibility	As handlers are the primary agent overseeing their dog's welfare, they must constantly make decisions around safeguarding their dog's well-being. This might include stopping a session to allow a dog to have a toilet break, illustrating how to obtain consent for a client, respecting a dog's decision to retreat from an interaction, and/or stopping a session entirely.
Social Awareness	– Perspective-taking – Empathy – Appreciating diversity – Respect for others	Strong perspective-taking skills are required by handlers as they support a variety of clients seeking to augment their well-being and decrease their ill-being through interactions with therapy dogs. Handlers too provide education to clients around how to interact with dogs.
Relationship Skills	– Communication – Social engagement – Relationship building – Teamwork	Handlers must first and foremost establish and maintain a healthy and supportive relationship with their dog. Next, we see handlers routinely meet and engage with members of the public.

Determining Dog-Handler Team Suitability for CAIs

of varied human clients. We might consider the therapy dog's *level of resiliency* – their ability to adapt to the demands placed on them – from their handler, from visiting clients, and from the contextual environment. The extent to which a therapy dog possesses temperament and behaviours known to contribute to successful CAIs, the more successful they'll be in not just adapting to the experience of working as a therapy dog but enjoying and thriving within sessions. Next, we examine the dispositions and behaviours that optimize a therapy dog's resiliency and ability to contribute to CAIs.

Dispositions

Recall that dispositions were defined earlier in this chapter as the natural qualities of character or temperament. More generally, we might consider the dispositions of therapy dogs as ranging from uptight and high strung to a demeanor that is flexible, relaxed, and calm. Having worked with hundreds of therapy dogs over the years, we know that although therapy dogs must be relaxed and calm, they must still be engaging. Dogs who are relaxed and calm but who have a flat or non-responsive personality can struggle to connect with clients. Next, we examine elements of temperament characterizing therapy dogs.

Responsive to Handler Commands

As handlers oversee and are responsible for their dog's behaviour and welfare, they must be able to manage and direct their dog in public. In turn, therapy dogs must respond consistently to the demands of their handlers. Take, for example, a handler who enters a facility to join a program and notices dropped food *en route* and gives their dog a "leave it" command. Here we see compliance with the handler's request key to safeguarding dog well-being. There are many behaviours expected of therapy dogs that are routine and do not require commands from handlers. This might include standing attentively for pre-session grooming, acceptance of a vest or wearing a form of identification, a loose-leash walk into facilities including passing through doorways or taking an elevator, stopping alongside the handler as the handler gathers information from program personnel (e.g., where to set up a station or position themselves to meet clients, the number of clients expected, etc.), and settling onto a comfort mat prior to the start of a session.

Dogs too will respond to direct commands from handlers, and within the context of CAIs, this may take the form of prompts. A common prompt used by handlers within a session is asking dogs "Who's this?" to alert dogs to a visitor and to allow the dog to sniff a lowered open palm to provide consent.

Secure Attachment to Handler

We've already addressed this in our discussions above; however, it merits repeating and nuancing here. In order for the therapy dog to welcome and engage visiting clients, there needs to be a foundational secure handler-dog attachment evident. It bears repeating here because we recognize and have seen that it's possible that the dog is insecurely attached to the handler despite the handler's wish for and attempts to establish healthy boundaries. Dogs who are insecurely attached to their handler may seek constant connection and reassurance through touch. In turn, these attention-seeking behaviours are likely to impede any engagement with clients, undermining both the handler's and the dog's ability to support clients.

Other Dog Indifference

Although dog-handler teams may work independently with one team visiting a location, oftentimes, given the demand to interact with therapy dogs, we see multiple teams volunteer together with dog-handler teams stationed side by side within a space. It is within such contexts that therapy dogs must be "other dog indifferent." A dog in this context who is focussed on greeting other dogs in the room will have a hard time connecting with clients as their attention is elsewhere and "other focussed." Clients undoubtedly would sense this, and the resultant interaction would be left wanting.

After years of overseeing programs, we have seen dog friendships develop over time (i.e., from the same dog-handler teams repeatedly attending the same sessions who cross paths in parking lots prior to the start of a session). In this case, consider allowing dogs to greet one another prior to settling. Not doing so can make settling challenging, and a simple sniff and hello between dogs so they can acknowledge each other can go a long way towards helping dogs feel comfortable. Bringing multiple dogs into the same space and not allowing them to greet one another is akin to humans attending a party but not being allowed to speak to anyone! Still, it is important that handlers recognize that a session where multiple dog-handler teams are volunteering concurrently is not a dog playdate opportunity where the purpose is to socialize dogs. Where interest in other dogs persists, we have found that a "ecological manipulation" of the dog-handler team can help reduce social temptations. This might include positioning the dog so their back is towards the other dog or having the entire dog-handler team station moved to the opposite side of the room.

Calm but Engaged

As a general rule, therapy dogs must be calm when in public where they are likely to encounter multiple stimuli; the combination of novel odors, other dogs, machinery, and multiple new people can collectively be exciting for dogs. When working in a CAI, therapy dogs are asked to cast aside all temptations to investigate these novelties and to remain calm in anticipation of meeting one or more clients. Added to this, therapy dogs should have a high startle reflex – they are not easily flustered by novelty and remain calm in the face of new stimuli (e.g., dropped crutches, announcements delivered via overhead speakers, heightened emotions from clients, etc.).

As an illustration of the importance of therapy dogs possessing a calm disposition, consider an excited client who is overcome with emotion at the mere sight of the therapy dog, recalling memories of their own dog back home and realizing, in the moment, how far they are from this source of love and support. Rather than the therapy dog rising to match this level of heightened excitement, the dog, in remaining calm, invites the client to join them in a calm state, quelling the client's heightened emotions.

Keen Curiosity to Meet the Public and Emotional Intuitiveness

As general dispositions, therapy dogs should be calm but engaged and attentive. They must have a genuine desire to meet new people and a certain curiosity about people in general. Recall the prompt described earlier that saw handlers engage their dog by saying "Who's this?" to

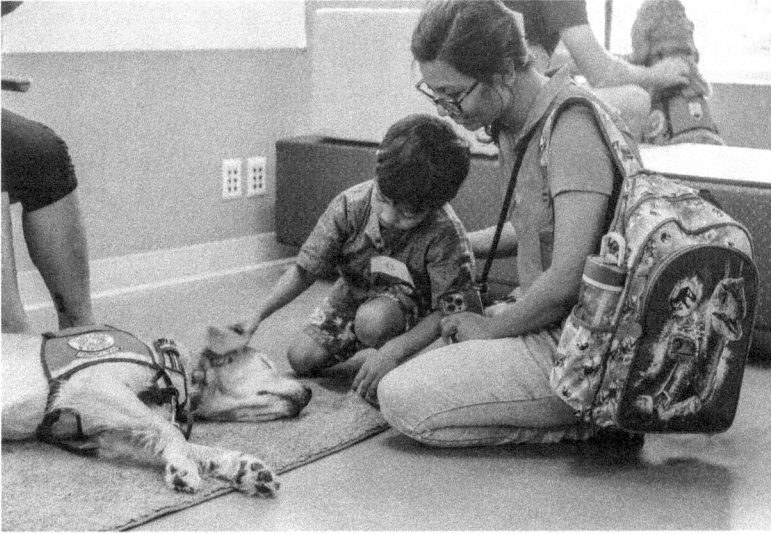

Figure 4.5 A parent oversees her child's interaction with therapy dog Baylee as he gently touches her ear. Baylee lies down on her comfort mat with her eyes closed

Source: Freya L. L. Green Photography; used with permission

announce a visitor to a session. The therapy dog should possess a keen desire to find out the answer to this question.

One thing that's guaranteed is that the clients taking part in a CAI will be varied on many dimensions, including the emotional profiles they bring to the session. In addition to clients of varied genders, races, dress codes, and behaviours, clients also arrive in varied emotional states. Recall our earlier discussions of emotional contagion – the passing of emotions from humans to the dogs and between humans. Therapy dogs with strong emotional intuition will sense the clients low in affect (i.e., heightened sadness) and may hone in on supporting these individuals over others who visit the station (Figure 4.5).

CONCLUSION

This chapter began with a scenario in which a handler was challenged by an interaction that compromised their dog's welfare – French fries fed to her dog. Threats to dog welfare like this are difficult to anticipate, but handlers who adopt a proactive approach (versus a reactive or corrective approach) optimize dog welfare by avoiding events that compromise welfare. Throughout this chapter, we elucidated the characteristics of both handlers and therapy dogs that help dog-handler teams optimally support clients in varied situations whilst upholding therapy dog welfare. Handlers play a key role in proactively managing their dog in public and creating an environment where therapy dogs can engage clients and perhaps even work intuitively, helping clients who need them most. We elucidated the different dispositions and skills required of handlers and used social and emotional competencies as a framework informing the skills needed by handlers. In Chapter 5 that follows, we examine, in detail, the factors that enhance and compromise dog-handler team welfare.

REFERENCES

Binfet, J. T., Draper, Z. A., & Green, F. L. L. (2020). Stress reduction in law enforcement officers and staff through a canine-assisted intervention. *Human–Animal Interaction Bulletin*, 8(2), 34–52. https://doi.org/10.1079/hai.2020.0011

Binfet, J. T., & Hartwig, E. (2020). *Canine-assisted interventions: A comprehensive guide to credentialing therapy dog teams*. Routledge. https://doi.org/10.4324/9780429436055

Collaborative for Academic and Social and Emotional Learning (2024; CASEL.org). Retrieved July 5 from: https://casel.org/fundamentals-of-sel/what-is-the-casel-framework/

Green, F. L. L., & Binfet, J. T. (2021). Therapy dogs, stress-reduction, and well-being within the detachment: Interviews with law-enforcement personnel. *Human–Animal Interaction Bulletin*, 11(1), 10–35. https://doi.org/10.1079/hai.2021.0018.

Oxford Learner's Dictionary (2024). *Disposition*. Retrieved July 5th from: https://www.oxfordlearnersdictionaries.com/definition/english/disposition

Pet Partners (2022). *Facility tool kit*. Retrieved June 12, 2024 from: https://petpartners.org/wp-content/uploads/2023/06/Facility-Toolkit_download-version.pdf

APPENDIX 4.1

Social and Emotional Competencies from the Collaborative for Academic and Social and Emotional Learning

(Image Source: ©2021 CASEL. All Rights Reserved. Used with permission. https://casel.org/fundamentals-of-sel/what-is-the-casel-framework/)

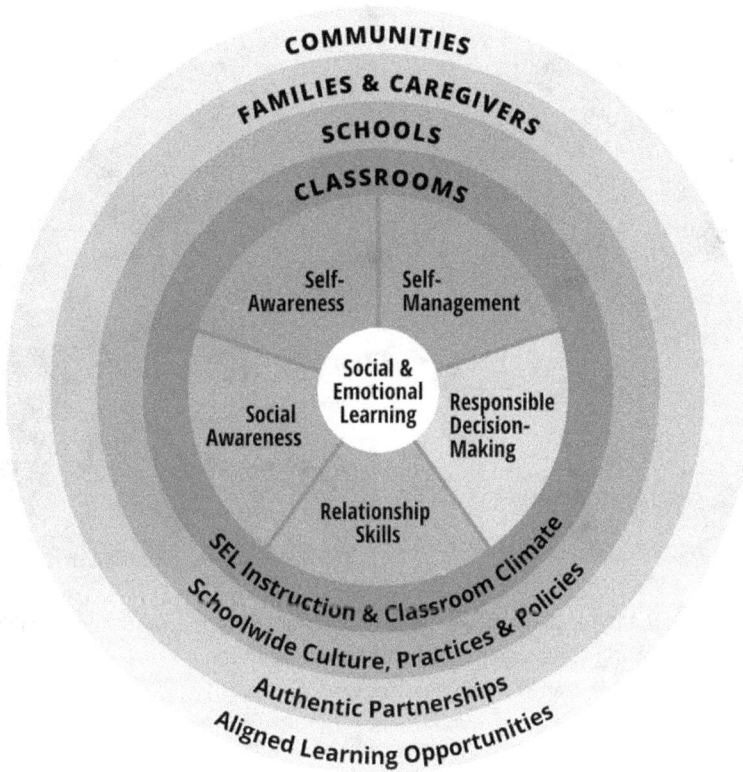

Five

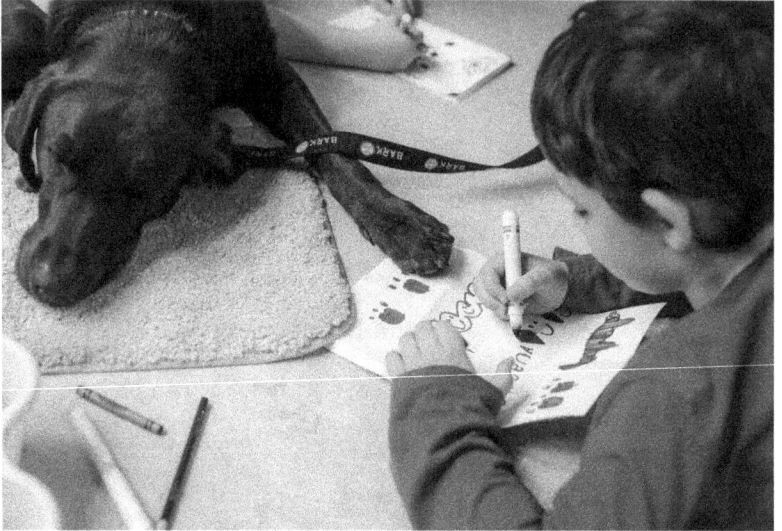

Figure 5.1 Therapy dog Skeena, a chocolate Labrador, rests comfortably while a young child lays nearby and draws a picture

Source: F. L. L. Green Photography; used with permission

DOI: 10.4324/9781032639284-5

SCENARIO

Therapy Dogs as Classmates – Building Social Connections Among Diverse Learners

Constance teaches at a local elementary school, and this year her fifth-grade classroom is diverse and includes several neurodivergent learners: one student who has autism, another student who has dyspraxia, and two students who have attention-deficit hyperactivity disorder. Constance is also a parent to a seven-year-old girl with dyspraxia, and she knows how children who are neurodiverse often face challenges in social situations at school; she finds it frustrating and heartbreaking to watch the students in her classroom who struggle with social interactions and friendships. She wants to do something to help her students make friends; thus, she arranges to have a therapy dog visitation one afternoon each week to facilitate social interactions and promote a sense of classroom community. The children in Constance's classroom are very excited when they get to visit with Miriam and Ezra, the handler-therapy dog team assigned to visit their classroom. Constance notices that, by the time they enter the classroom, the children are shrieking with laughter, bouncing in their desk seats, and barely able to contain their excitement! They simultaneously jostle to reach Miriam and Ezra and compete for the dog's attention by calling out her name and whistling. Still, one student tries to lie on top of the therapy dog while stroking her firmly on the head. Another student inadvertently places his hand inside the therapy dog's mouth, and this clearly startles the dog. Constance didn't expect the children's dynamic and unique reactions. It's obvious to Constance that Miriam and Ezra are fostering joyful social interactions among all the children in her classroom, but she also observes that Miriam, the dog handler, appears anxious and she later learns that Miriam is concerned that Ezra is distressed by the student's excitement. Constance is dismayed to hear that Miriam is reconsidering her weekly visit with Ezra. Not wanting to disappoint her students, Constance asks Miriam to brainstorm ways that they can better prepare to facilitate a more mutually rewarding visitation between her diverse students and the dog-handler team (Figure 5.1).

QUESTIONS FOR REFLECTION AND DISCUSSION

1. How should therapy dog sessions in dynamic applied contexts be structured? Where should sessions unfold and how much supervision should they involve? How long should sessions last?

2. What special considerations should a handler and educator be required to receive prior to introducing students to a therapy dog in applied and dynamic contexts? Should a handler be required to receive training before engaging therapy dogs in their practice with neurodivergent learners?

3. What guidance should neurodivergent learners receive in advance of meeting a dog-handler team? Should the handler or educator be responsible for educating learners about how to interact with therapy dogs? Should a handler collect information about the learner's past experiences with animals?

4. How might we assess if the session is rewarding for both the learner and the therapy dog? What indicators should an educator consider?

5. To optimize therapy dog welfare in applied dynamic contexts, what conditions should be in place for therapy dogs? What conditions should be in place within sessions involving diverse learners?

DYNAMIC APPLIED CONTEXTS AND DOG-HANDLER TEAM WELFARE

... contrary to disappointing clients, privileging animal agency and autonomy models a foundation of compassion and caring that can only strengthen the handler/client relationship.

(Townsend & Gee, 2021, p. 14)

This scenario illustrates a typical situation in elementary classrooms where a group of diverse students simultaneously and uniquely express their enthusiasm to engage with therapy dogs. Despite a teacher's best intentions, if the students' enthusiasm is not properly managed, it can create stress for the dog-handler team and compromise the dog's enjoyment of the session. In previous chapters, we have learned that many canine-assisted interventions (CAIs) unfold casually and informally and within dynamic applied contexts. In this chapter, we consider how dynamic applied contexts present a whole host of potential threats to the welfare of both the therapy dog and the handler; inherently, these settings are characterized by complex and often unpredictable contingencies that can shape therapy dogs' experiences of stress and handlers' ability to advocate for their dog's welfare. We aim to create awareness around factors potentially undermining a dog-handler team's welfare and ability to support human clients and consider factors that both compromise and enhance therapy dogs and their handlers when CAIs are delivered in dynamic applied settings. This discussion will be valued by educators such as Constance, the teacher in our opening scenario, who aim to structure and facilitate successful interactions between their diverse students and therapy dog-handler teams.

INDICATORS OF COMPROMISED DOG AND HANDLER WELFARE

As can be imagined, there is no shortage of potential obstacles or challenges that individually and collectively can undermine and thwart the welfare of both the handler and therapy dogs participating in CAIs. We begin with an overview of some of the indicators of compromised dog and handler welfare in CAIs before turning our attention to some of the factors undermining and enhancing therapy dog-handler team welfare (see Figure 5.2). First, we consider some of the physical, behavioural, and emotional indicators of canine stress in the context of CAIs, and then we discuss some indicators of handler stress during CAIs. We also provide an ethogram of canine stress signals (see Table 5.1) and a checklist (see Table 5.2) for readers, offering them support and guidance in the creation and actualization of CAIs.

Signs of Canine Stress

Importantly, researchers suggest that participating in CAIs may prove stressful for some therapy dogs (e.g., Fatjó et al., 2021; Sarrafchi et al., 2022; Silas et al., 2019; Uccheddu et al., 2018). Stress signals are unique to every therapy dog, ranging from subtle to obvious, and varying across CAI contexts and clients (for reviews, see Ng, 2021; Provoost, 2021; Townsend & Gee, 2021). Shepherd has proposed a ladder of dog behaviours that indicate increasing levels of stress (Shepherd, 2002), and, more recently, McCullough and colleagues (2018; see Table 5.1)

Table 5.1 Canine Behaviour Ethogram

Behaviour	Description	How to Score
Affiliative Indicators		
Leaning or resting body or head against a person or object	Leaning or resting body or head against a person or object	Count each time the dog leans or puts head down. If dog moves away, then replaces head or leans again, count again. Dog is seeking contact, not just resting.
Licking a person	Passing the tongue over any part of the person's body	Count each period of licking, i.e., if multiple licks over and over, just count once. Then if dog stops licking and starts again, count again.
Pawing/paw lifting	Forearm lifted to a 45-degree angle; paw extended or "waved"; sometimes paw touches the person	Count each time paw is lifted. If dog puts paw down and then lifts again, count again. Dog is seeking attention.
Play stance/bow	Excited and alert affect; bottom raised; tail raised and wagging; front of body lowered; front knees bent; tongue out; head forward and erect; ears perked up; eyes wide and bright; dog may jump around and vocalize in anticipation	Count each time the dog bows.
Pushing snout/ seeking pet	Pushing, investigating, or eliciting contact with the snout at any body part of the person; "goosing," shoving, or poking a person (usually the handler or someone familiar to the dog)	This is typically a dog nosing a person's hand for petting. Count once for each time the dog "asks" for more petting.
Raising ears (breed-specific)	Ears noticeably raise or perk up	This could be in response to seeing a person, hearing an interesting noise, or responding to the person calling the dog or squeaking a toy. The dog is showing friendly interest. Count once for each time the dog perks his ears.

Behaviour	Description	How to Score
Rolling over	Rolling over on back, exposing abdomen; may be accompanied with body or limb stretching and/or self-directed behaviours (e.g., scratching)	Although this behaviour can be either stress related or affiliative, typically a therapy dog will roll over to seek petting. Count once for each time the dog rolls over.
Tail wagging	Tail moves repeatedly side to side or up and down	Count once for each period of tail wagging. If tail stops wagging but then resumes, count again.
Walking/approach	Walking forward; walking towards a person	Count once for each time the dog approaches the client. This will likely be just upon entrance.
Moderate Stress Indicators		
Body shaking or "shaking off"	Body shaking or trembling involuntarily OR "shaking off" voluntarily (like when wet or dirty)	May happen after being hugged or close contact. Count once for each shaking episode.
Escape	Efforts to get away from the eliciting stimulus by pulling on leash, backing up, hiding behind handler, digging, etc.	May signal the dog is done visiting – tries to get off the bed and/or walks away from the client (e.g., away from client, towards the door). Count once each time the dog initiates the motion.
Looking at/to handler	Frequent looking at/ to handler during interaction with client/ patient; gazing at handler during interaction	Dog seems unsure of what they are supposed to do – looks to the handler for guidance or direction. Count once for each time the dog looks up/at the handler.
Looking away	Head turning away from the person; averting eyes/gaze from the person	The dog purposefully turns away from the client who may be trying to get close to the dog's face. Count once each time the dog turns their head.
Oral behaviours/ lip licking	Tongue out; tongue briefly extended; lip licking; snout/ nose licking; floor licking; swallowing; lip smacking	Count once when you see the dog's tongue extend from their mouth. Count as a licking period – not each individual lick. For each period of five licks or more, count as one period of licking.

(continued)

Table 5.1 (Cont.)

Behaviour	Description	How to Score
Panting – excessive or prolonged	Breathing quickly or in a labored fashion; tongue usually out; abdomen may noticeably move up and down	Count once for each panting period. If the dog stops and resumes, count again.
Restlessness	Frequent changes in posture or position; frequent "changes in the state of locomotion"; circling; difficulty sitting or lying still	Seems the dog needs to readjust position – may be physically uncomfortable. Could be coupled with trying to leave the bed/room and move towards the door. Count once each time the motion occurs.
Self-directed behaviours	Grooming; scratching; licking; biting; chewing	The dog interrupts visiting with the client to chew/scratch on self. Count once for each chewing/licking/scratching episode.
Yawning	Open mouth; inhalation of breath/air followed quickly by exhalation	Count once each time you see the dog yawn unless it's a repetitive period.
High Stress Indicators		
Baring teeth	Pulling the upper lips up and back so the teeth are visible (lip "curling"); snarling	Typically paired with growling, looking as if the dog will bite.
Barking, yelping, yipping, whining, or whimpering	Relatively brief vocalizations of varying pitch without growly undertones	Not "talking" on command or vocalizing for attention – aggressive or stressed/unhappy vocalizations.
Biting or attempting to bite	Mouth open; teeth exposed; head forward; clamping (or attempting to clamp) the skin of a person between the jaws; may cause noticeable wound on a person who is bitten	Different than mouthing during play – aggressive action against patient or others.
Crouching	Body crouched low; legs bent; bottom and head lowered; back arched; tail may be between hind legs; cowering	The dog is/looks backed into a corner and does not want a person to approach.

Behaviour	Description	How to Score
Drooling – excessive or in copious amounts	Increased salivation or moisture around the nose and mouth	Not food-induced – unusual or excessive drooling.
Ears plastered/ pinned back	Ears positioned lower and/or backward (in response to stimulus)	Sometimes paired with a submissive approach and may be followed by rolling over.
Growling	A throaty and rumbling vocalization, usually low in pitch	The dog makes a "warning" sound that they feel protective/stressed.
Stare gaze	An intense, fixed, and direct gaze into the eyes of the person; eyes may be dilated or the whites of the eyes may be clearly visible	Part of a prey instinct – the dog looks as if they are hunting.

Source: McCullough et al., 2018; used with permission from *Applied Animal Behavior Science*

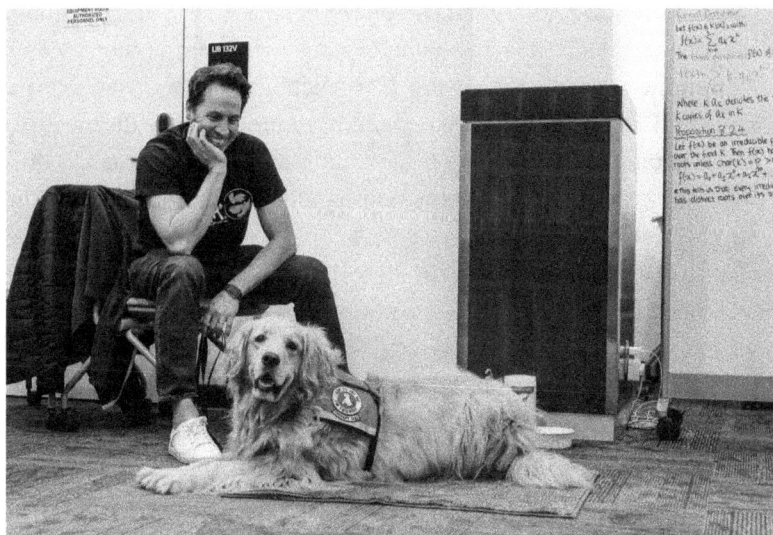

Figure 5.2 Therapy dog-handler team Warren and Ollie smiling and sharing a positive emotional experience as they await clients. Ollie is settled at his station and in a relaxed lie-down position.

Source: F. L. L. Green Photography; used with permission

have outlined detailed guidelines to assess affiliative indicators and behavioural indicators of moderate and high stress in therapy dogs. To begin, subtle and milder, physical indicators of canine stress include paw lifting and lip licking and turning away from human contact or involvement in a CAI-related activity. Whereas more salient and harsher, physical indicators of canine stress include growling, snapping, or biting. Clearly, a therapy dog that is enjoying their involvement in a CAI will show a relaxed posture, open mouth, and movement towards rather than away from an interaction or specific activity (Townsend & Gee, 2021). Other behavioural indicators of canine distress include whether the therapy dog is showing signs of avoidance and displacement (e.g., looking away, hiding, leaning against handler, yawning, or sniffing), fear (e.g., lowering head, tucking tail, flattening ears, or bracing hind legs), problematic eye gazing (e.g., directed gazing or looking away; gazing pattern is deemed unusual for the specific dog), freezing (e.g., postures that minimize visibility, difficulty responding to handler's directions), or aggression (e.g., raised hackles, closed mouth, staring, and emotional and behavioural alertness and readiness for action). Relatedly, it is important to assess whether the therapy dog is communicating dissent during CAIs such as moving away from a human-initiated interaction or remaining motionless and disengaged. In the section that follows, we discuss the importance of therapy dog consent to the welfare of therapy dog-handler teams and their ability to support human clients.

As noted above, stress experiences are unique to each therapy dog and may vary widely as a function of additional factors including a therapy dog's age, fatigue, and physical health. Therapy dog welfare might also be compromised by the stress they experience from various aspects of their involvement in CAIs, such as the proximity of other animals, particularly for dogs who do not show "other dog indifference" as discussed in Chapter 4. Other aspects of therapy dogs' involvement in CAIs that can contribute to stress and reduced welfare include adjusting to new environments, managing different types and sizes of clients, and the duration and intensity of their sessions. For instance, older therapy dogs might become fatigued more easily when participating in CAIs, despite having greater familiarity with the context; they might show greater enjoyment (or boredom, a possible stressor) when participating in a CAI. Younger dogs, in contrast, might show less fatigue, but increased stress or overstimulation (or enjoyment) when engaging in novel CAI-related activities. Indeed, in one study, stress-related behaviours (e.g., panting, licking) were more frequently noted in younger therapy dogs and in dogs with less therapy experience after they participated in a hospital-based therapy session (King et al., 2011). Further, therapy dogs might become more easily fatigued (cognitively and emotionally) when experiencing physical illness or by participating in CAI sessions that are lengthy, involve several clients or a steady rotation of clients, or involve intense human emotions. Handlers may want to consider if their dog enjoys interacting with a small number of clients in a group setting or one-on-one in a more intimate setting.

Handlers should also consider their dog's unique energy levels and preferences in terms of contextual stimuli and human interaction. For instance, does their dog have experience with loud noises and quickly moving objects? Does their dog have experience with humans expressing intense emotions? Does their dog enjoy being touched by several people and, if so, for what length of time? Does their dog show a preference for personal space? Does their dog enjoy mentally and physically stimulating activities or simple and relaxing activities? What type of client does their dog enjoy spending time with – active, quiet, excitable, or tranquil clients? Does their dog enjoy interacting with children, youth, or senior clients? Each of these variables and contexts holds the potential to create undue stress for a therapy dog depending on their unique experiences, preferences, and energy levels; handlers have a responsibility to consider these factors prior to involving their dogs in a CAI. Here the goal is to engage each therapy dog in a CAI that offers an enriching and rewarding experience – a CAI context that represents a *goodness of fit* between therapy dog and environment (VanFleet, 2014). Recall the scenario at the outset of this chapter, Constance's classroom would have been an ideal CAI context for a therapy dog who enjoys being touched and spending time with a group of diverse and excitable children and who possesses a certain adaptability and *level of resiliency*. As discussed in Chapter 4, a therapy dog who shows these preferences and characteristics is likely to better adapt to the demands placed on them within CAI sessions including expressions of intense emotions, diverse communication and mobility patterns, quickly moving objects, and loud noises. Perhaps more important, such a therapy dog might enjoy and thrive within CAI sessions unfolding within Constance's classroom – there would be a *goodness of fit* between therapy dog and environment.

Further, veterinarians highlight trigger-loading as an important contributor to canine stress (Overall, 2013). Also known as *trigger-stacking*, trigger-loading occurs when a dog experiences multiple stressors without an opportunity to return to a baseline state of calm; the dog's stress/arousal level remains heightened. For instance, when a therapy dog participates in several novel experiences "stacked up" one after the other leading up to a CAI session, without adequate rest in between, they might experience increased arousal/stress and exhibit unpredictable behaviours (Overall, 2013). Here, it is important to note that trigger-stacking stress experiences and stress signalling can differ for each dog. This variability underscores the need for handlers to have intimate knowledge of their therapy dog's unique stress-related experiences and signalling patterns. Further, handlers' knowledge about their dogs must be put into practice within highly dynamic applied contexts often characterized by complex and unpredictable contingencies as they advocate for their dog's welfare. In Chapter 6, we discuss further the varied contexts in which CAIs unfold and the many real-time challenges that handlers can face when assessing and handling their therapy dog's stress, despite knowing their dogs intimately and their best intentions to safeguard their dog's welfare.

Signs of Handler Stress

The role of handlers in CAIs should not be underestimated. Just as stress signals are unique to every therapy dog, so too are indicators of stress among human handlers – both can vary widely within the context of CAIs (for discussions, see Binfet & Hartwig, 2020; Tardif-Williams & Binfet, 2023). Stressed handlers might fail to engage clients by asking questions and inviting and facilitating interactions with the therapy dog. Handlers who are stressed might fail to make eye contact with clients, interact minimally and quietly, and engage in abrupt verbal exchanges with clients. Still, a handler who is feeling unsure about their own and their dog's participation in a CAI might exhibit signs of protectiveness by holding tightly to the therapy dog's leash; this can restrict the dog's movement and the client's access to the dog. As we've acknowledged in our discussion of emotional contagion, the handler's apprehension here could negatively impact the emotional state of their dog as well.

Several factors and challenges can contribute to handler stress and undermine handler welfare while participating in CAIs. Handlers' years of experience participating in CAIs can contribute to feelings of stress, as novice handlers (like their therapy dogs) might become more easily fatigued when engaging in novel CAI-related activities while managing their dog's behaviour and monitoring welfare. In this way, novice versus more experienced handlers may overlook stress signalling in their dogs. Just as therapy dogs might become more easily fatigued (cognitively and emotionally) by CAI sessions that are too lengthy, involve a steady rotation of clients, or are characterized by intense human emotions, so too can handlers become fatigued and/or stressed under such conditions. Handler preferences, energy levels, and enjoyment of CAIs must also be considered; handlers should consider the types of clients and session activities they enjoy, and if they enjoy working with a small number of clients in a group setting or one-on-one in a more intimate setting. It merits noting that, as is the case with therapy dogs, there should be a *goodness* of fit between the handler and CAI context. Both therapy dog and handler welfare and enjoyment must be optimized during CAIs. We suggest that handlers who comfortably enjoy their participation in CAIs are better able to advocate for their dog's welfare and the dog-handler team is better able to support human clients.

Further, sometimes handlers' capacity to advocate for their dog can be hampered by social desirability – handlers are apt to want their dog to work and offer a supportive interaction for the clients. For instance, an enthusiastic handler might hide their dog's restlessness from the program staff because they want to be perceived as a competent and supportive therapy dog-handler team. Also, handlers might also enjoy the interactions involved in CAIs and be inclined to hold a biased perception that their therapy dog enjoys these interactions as much as they or the clients do (Ng et al., 2015). Both social desirability and biased perceptions might lead to oversights in dog welfare during CAIs, and handlers may not want to draw attention to their dog's welfare concerns because they worry about possible reprisals from therapy dog organizations or that their participation in CAIs will be terminated. Handlers might also be sensitive to disappointing clients and continue with CAI activities even though their dog might be showing signs of fatigue or overwork; well-intentioned handlers might be inclined to overlook their dog's signs of stress in favour of supporting the clients.

Handlers might also perceive pressure to continue with CAI activities from other agents including teachers, clinicians, or hospital staff who have invested time, space, and resources to support CAIs. In the scenario described at the beginning of this chapter, the handler, Miriam, might feel pressured from the teacher, Constance, and the students to continue the CAI session with Ezra, her therapy dog. As a result, she might continue the session for longer than she feels comfortable and might overlook or be less inclined to respond to Ezra's stress signalling.

Additionally, it warrants mention that handlers play a *bifurcated* or *split role* in the context of CAIs; this is a unique and sometimes challenging role (Glenk & Foltin, 2021). In a study by Colleen Dell and colleagues (2021), participants (handlers) noted that the handler serves as a translator between the client and the dog and described the handler as a "connection to the dog" (p. 4). They also described their bifurcated role as being pulled in two directions and as taxing and very draining, as they must manage their dog's interactions and monitor their dog's welfare, all the while supporting the client. Ng and colleagues (2015) argue that animal welfare in animal-assisted interventions should be continuously assessed to determine animal stress and fatigue. Ideally, as discussed in Chapter 3, it would be helpful to have a person dedicated solely to monitoring therapy dog welfare in CAIs; however, this is not always feasible as CAIs are sometimes carried out informally and with few resources. Here, we position the handler as the ideal person to undertake this responsibility as they work alongside their dog to deliver CAIs and have intimate knowledge of their dog's typical behaviours and preferences. In this way, handlers play a unique role and hold a large responsibility in the context of CAIs. Handlers also recognize their role as advocates for their dog's welfare in CAIs. In a qualitative study involving online surveys with 111 French therapy dog handlers, handlers positioned themselves as the ultimate gatekeeper of therapy dog welfare in the context of CAIs and highlighted their responsibility as advocates for optimizing dog welfare (Mignot et al., 2022). Therefore, we recommend that handlers be prepared in advance for the demands that will be placed on them and their therapy dog when participating in CAIs. Such preparation can allow handlers to focus their attention more fully on assessing their dog's welfare and enjoyment in CAIs. Ng and Fine (2021) offer a useful behavioural instrument for assessing and scoring therapy dog welfare before, during, and following a CAI session (see Table 5.2).

Table 5.2 Pet-Assisted Therapy Welfare Tool

Behavioral parameters		Score	Result
Aggression	No sign of aggression	0	
	Growling or barking when interacting with people, strong eye contact	1	
	Lunging toward or attempting to bite people	2	
	Biting people	3	
Fear/Anxiety/ Stress	No sign of fear, anxiety, or stress	0	
	Licks lips/nose, excessive salivation, pawing, tail between legs, no eye contact	1	
	Crouching both standing and sitting, whining, shaking, restless, agitated, yawning	2	
	Cowering, "whale eye," attempting to escape from situation	3	
Excitability	Calm, no signs of being overly excited	0	
	Increased alertness, nose, ears, and tail up, curious about something or event	1	
	Yelping. frequent change in posture, rushing toward exciting thing or event	2	
	Hard to calm down even when exciting thing or event are removed	3	
Interaction with people	Greets people without hesitation, tail wags at backlevel, accepts treats	0	
	Mild encouragement needed to interact with person, hesitant sniffing	1	
	Allows petting, but backs away quickly, accepts treats thrown away from person	2	
	Will not approach with encouragement, avoids interaction, does not take treats	3	
Interaction with dogs	Ignores other dogs present in the vicinity of the therapy session	0	
	Distracted by the presence of other dogs	1	
	Directs attention to other dogs and/or tries to interact with them	2	
	Attacks other dogs or barks at them	3	
Obedience	Obeys commands quickly	0	
	Hesitates to obey or performs behavior only briefly, licks lips, yawns, scratches	1	

(continued)

Table 5.2 (Cont.)

Behavioral parameters		Score	Result
	Strong encouragement needed to perform, whines, avoids eye contact	2	
	Ignores handler completely	3	
Tiredness	Looks fresh and active. Wants to join in therapy session	0	
	Only joins if activities are really engaging	1	
	Prefers to stay quiet and is uninterested	2	
	Does not move. Prefers to lie down. Does not take rewards	3	
Reactivity	Does not react at all to loud noise or sudden and strange movements	0	
	Moves slightly when strange stimuli appear (loud noise, sudden movement, etc.)	1	
	Jumps or barks when strange stimuli appear (loud noise, sudden movement, etc.)	2	
	Runs or jumps on people when strange stimuli appear (loud noise, sudden movement, etc.)	3	
Anticipation	No special behavior before changing activity (e.g., entering the AAT space)	0	
	Licks lips or nose, excessive salivation, pawing, tail between legs, no eye contact before changing activity (e.g., entering the AAT space)	1	
	Avoids entering a known place (e.g., the AAT space)	2	
	Runs away or vocalizes before changing activity (e.g., entering the AAT space)	3	
Scoring factor	If the score is 3 more than once, add an extra point for each score=3	2	
		3	
		4	
		5	
		6	
		7	
	Total score		
Instructions	For each parameter, write down the appropriate score in the RESULT column and then calculate the sum of all scores		

(continued)

Table 5.2 (Cont.)

Behavioral parameters		Score	Result
	Write down the score if any of the behaviors are present. For example, any sign of fear would beat least "1." It is not necessary that the dog displays all behaviors in the list at once		
	Based on the total score take the appropriate actions based on the total score:		
0-10=	Well-being is generally acceptable. The dog shows no clear sign of being affected by her/his involvement in the therapy session and no special measures need to be taken		
11-15=	Well-being may start to be affected. Observe the dog more carefully and consider removing the animal from the session and providing some time to rest away from other people and animals		
16-24=	Well-being impact is more serious. Dog should be removed from the specific activity and given an opportunity to rest and relax. Before using the animal again, Welfare Assessment Instrument should be applied again to make sure that the score has lowered		
>25=	Well-being is severely affected. Dog should be immediately removed from the specific activity and placed in an environment that allows for supervision without interfering with the ability of the dog to recover. If this occurs more than once, serious consideration should be given to the suitability of the dog as a therapy animal. A third party with experience in animal welfare assessments, for example, a veterinarian or an animal behaviorist, should be consulted before the animal is used again for a more professional assessment		

Source: Peralta & Fine, 2021; used with permission from Springer

In addition to attending to the therapy dog's welfare and enjoyment in CAIs, consideration should be given to optimizing the handler's welfare and enjoyment as they too are key agents in making CAIs successful for supporting human clients.

FACTORS ENHANCING DOG AND HANDLER WELFARE

Building on our discussion of canine and handler stress indicators and some of the factors compromising dog and handler welfare in CAIs, we now turn our attention to some of the variables and conditions that help to optimize dog-handler team welfare and their ability to support human clients. This includes a critical discussion of therapy dog enjoyment and agency, the handler as an educator and advocate, the importance of client education, and a focus on understanding the importance of, and how to execute, the concept of therapy dog consent. We also provide a checklist for readers, offering them support and guidance in the creation and actualization of CAIs (see Table 5.2).

Attending to Therapy Dog Welfare and Enjoyment and Agency in CAIs
Recent research highlights the nuanced cognitive and emotional lives of animals. In this way, similar to their human handlers, therapy dogs can experience both the advantages and disadvantages of their therapeutic roles within CAIs (for a discussion, see Peralta & Fine, 2021). Recent research aims to better understand therapy dogs' experiences and affective states during CAIs; participating in CAIs can be stressful for therapy dogs (see Fatjó et al., 2021; Hatch, 2007; Sarrafchi et al., 2022; Silas et al., 2019). Therapy dogs' welfare and enjoyment during CAIs are integral in making CAIs successful in supporting human clients. Therefore, while we must take care to meet therapy dogs' basic needs during CAIs, consideration should also be extended to the emotional and cognitive welfare of therapy dogs during CAIs – greater attention must be given to how the *dog experiences* the CAI environment (Enders-Slegers, 2019; Glenk, 2017; Peralta & Fine, 2021; Winkle & Johnson Binder, 2024). Indeed, as in humans, we can glean much about therapy dogs' affective states during CAIs by assessing behavioural markers and measuring cortisol and other physiologic parameters such as heart rate and heart rate variability (for reviews, see Ng, 2021; Novack et al., 2023; Winkle et al., 2020).

In the context of CAIs, therapy dogs should be given an opportunity to experience positive emotional states, agency, and autonomy. Practically, we must consider the therapy dog's enjoyment and willingness to participate in CAIs. We must ask, "Does the therapy dog enjoy interacting with this particular group of clients?", "Is the therapy dog willing to engage with the client in a specific CAI context"? These considerations are in concert with The International Association of Human-Animal Interaction Organizations's commitment to ensuring that animal-assisted activities "should only be performed with the assistance of animals that are in good health, both physically and emotionally and that enjoy this type of activity" (Jegatheesan et al., 2019). Researchers also highlight the importance of *canine enrichment* activities (e.g., diverse, and novel social and sensory experiences) in increasing therapy dogs' enjoyment of CAIs (Townsend & Gee, 2021). As noted previously, we must consider if there is a *goodness of fit* between CAI activities and each therapy dog's temperament, preferences for human touch and contact, and energy level. CAI sessions should be structured

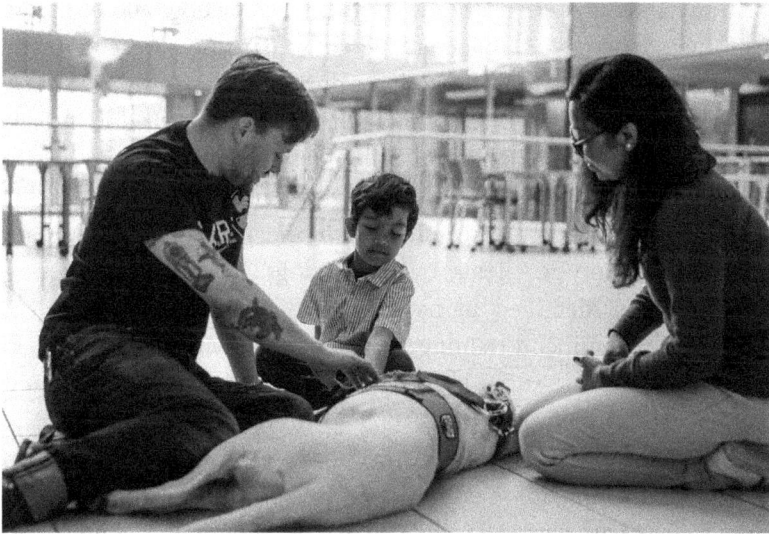

Figure 5.3 Therapy dog Dewey rests comfortably while a child sits nearby with his guardian and receives instruction from handler Michael on how to gently touch a dog
Source: F. L. L. Green Photography; used with permission

to respect therapy dogs' dignity, preferences, and enjoyment of their role as partners. Therapy dogs should also be able to experience a degree of agency in their roles within the CAI context – that is, they should have *genuine choice* or the *ability to choose* if they prefer to engage with clients (Novack et al., 2023). To be clear, therapy dogs should be *free* or independent to perform a range of normal behaviours including choosing to move away from clients or walking out of a room altogether (Mellor, 2016; Spinka, 2019). We discuss the practical application of therapy dog agency and consent within the context of CAIs in a later section. These considerations to optimizing therapy dog welfare within the context of CAIs are in alignment with the definition of therapy dog welfare we proffered in Chapter 3 and which we elaborate throughout this book.

THE ROLE OF HANDLER AS EDUCATOR AND ADVOCATE

It is one thing to identify factors that compromise therapy dog welfare in CAIs, but it is important to identify the people responsible for monitoring and verifying therapy dog welfare during CAIs. Here, we position handlers as key advocates for their therapy dogs and overseers ensuring the successful implementation of welfare measures to support their dog's participation and welfare during CAIs (Gee, 2023; Ng, 2021). Handlers are well positioned to advocate for their dog in CAIs by establishing what Winkle and colleagues (2020) refer to as *rules of engagement* which prioritize their dog's preferences for various aspects of CAIs including type of client, length and type of activities, and physical proximity to clients and other dogs. However, considering the challenges identified in handlers' bifurcated role (Dell et al., 2021), we recommend training or practice sessions where handlers and their therapy dogs can become familiar with the procedures and expectations in delivering CAIs to help mitigate welfare risks (Ng, 2021). Training and practice or simulation sessions would also help ensure that therapy dog-handler teams are comfortable and can optimally engage with clients. In addition, having program personnel who can assist with clients and monitor therapy dog welfare can reduce the burden of tasks on the shoulders of the handler and help ensure therapy dog welfare during CAI sessions. To ensure implementation fidelity and optimize both therapy dog and handler welfare, we also recommend having both new and seasoned handlers use a script and follow specific protocols to engage a range of clients and participants. New handlers, especially, may welcome training and practice sessions involving a script and protocol for engaging clients (Figure 5.3).

Further, as Winkle and Johnson Binder (2024) argue, owners/handlers should have at least an intermediate-level understanding of individual dog traits and preferences, behaviours, and training prior to including a dog in an animal-assisted intervention. It is critical that handlers receive training and practice in identifying canine stress signals. Research shows, however, that there is a lack of knowledge about canine stress signals among people more generally, including children and adults (Meints et al., 2018). Still, studies show that dog owners, and handlers, can often miss subtle signs of canine stress even in their own dogs (Mariti et al., 2012) for reasons related to aspects of both the handler (e.g., familiarity with a specific dog) and the dog (e.g., dog's individual expressions of distress). As such, it is critical that handlers and program personnel involved in CAIs receive training on how to identify subtle and early signs of canine stress. Relatedly, handlers should be able to identify signs of illness in their therapy dog which might contribute to compromised welfare in the context of CAIs; the complicated issue of when it is in the best interest of the therapy dog to retire must also be considered (for a discussion, see Ng & Fine, 2071).

The Importance of Client Education

It merits noting that welfare risks can be mitigated through educating and instructing visiting clients on how to optimally interact with therapy dogs. This important component of CAIs is often overseen by handlers and, in some cases, program personnel and is vital to optimizing therapy dog welfare and enjoyment. Ideally, clients would receive this education and instruction in advance of a session; however, it is often the case that clients will spontaneously attend sessions delivered in public venues without prior registration and/or there is little advance notice that a group of clients will be participating in a session. This lack of pre-planning makes it challenging for handlers to take proactive steps to instruct clients on how best to interact with their therapy dog in advance of a session (recognizing that the greater the client is educated and informed about how best to interact during a session, the greater the dogs, welfare is protected and optimized). Further, the stresses of their bifurcated role might mean that handlers must juggle meeting the client's needs while monitoring and advocating for their therapy dog's welfare. Returning to the scenario at the outset of this chapter, Constance and Miriam should consult in advance to educate and instruct the students on how best to interact with Ezra to optimize Ezra's welfare, agency, positive affect, and enjoyment throughout the session. As an example, in one study evaluating a canine welfare education intervention, children (aged eight to nine years) in the intervention group showed significant pre- to post-test improvements in canine emotion recognition as compared to children in the control group; children's canine recognition is an important skill and a key therapy dog welfare consideration in CAIs (Iqbal et al., 2023). The students in Constance's classroom should also learn about therapy dog consent (see the next section) in advance of the first visit, and efforts should be made to teach them about how to optimally interact with Ezra to emphasize principles of mutual respect and maximize their shared enjoyment.

ENSURING CANINE CONSENT

I recommend that researchers and handlers be mindful of the animal's perspectives of the activities they are engaging in; strive not just for lack of poor welfare but also the presence of positive welfare; and work towards standards of affirmative consent.

(Horowitz, 2021, p. 5)

As discussed in Chapter 3, researchers and practitioners are shining a light on therapy dog agency and consent during CAIs. Questions to consider in the practical application of therapy dog agency and consent include: What it means? How it should be ascertained and by whom? And whether it should be assessed at one point in time or continuously? To be sure, handlers hold the responsibility of ensuring that their dog's agency, preferences for human touch and contact, and enjoyment are respected throughout CAIs. It is critical that handlers attend to their dog's agency and consent in CAIs as it holds implications for the quality of their shared relationship and the work

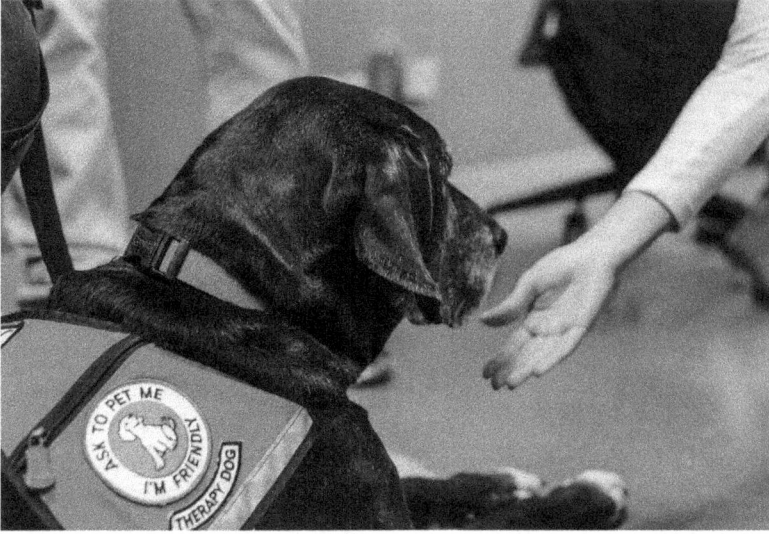

Figure 5.4 A hand is reaching out towards therapy dog Layla's chest requesting her consent to be touched

Source: F. L. L. Green Photography; used with permission

they undertake as a team (Iannuzzi & Rowan, 1991). Handlers can advocate for their dog by teaching people how to approach them and how to optimally interact with them (Figure 5.4).

Handlers can also pay close attention to their dog's body language and behaviour, noting if their dog appears to move towards or away from people's attempts to make physical contact with their dog. An important way to respect therapy dogs' agency during CAIs is to ascertain if they are willing participants by conducting a *consent-to-pet-test*. In the context of a CAIs, a canine consent test could involve having a potential participant adopt a sideways and non-threatening stance while holding an open palm near the therapy dog's chest. If the therapy dog remains motionless or moves away, then this would indicate their *dissent* or unwillingness to being touched. However, if the therapy dog moves towards the palm and initiates physical contact, then this would indicate their willingness or *consent* to being touched. Ideally, *consent-to-pet tests* should be carried out prior to each CAI session involving new clients and novel contexts as shifts in client and environmental characteristics might contribute to therapy dog stress. Further, to ensure the safety of both therapy dogs and clients in CAIs,

Winkle and colleagues (2020) suggest that consent tests should first be administered by competent adults or handlers who are unfamiliar with the dog. Returning to the scenario at the outset of this chapter, Constance should teach her classroom of diverse students about how best to approach a dog and ask the dog for consent to be touched. This could take the form of a lesson plan prior to receiving a visit from Miriam and Ezra and would help prepare the students for a more successful CAI session, one that would respect Ezra's agency and prioritize their shared enjoyment of the session.

Further, in one study, researchers found that canine salivary cortisol concentrations were higher on therapy days than on non-therapy days and were higher following therapy sessions of shorter duration (Haubenhofer & Kirchengast, 2006). Considering this latter finding, and the knowledge that therapy dogs differ in their response to a variety of stressors, handlers should know their dogs well and be especially mindful of their dog's willingness to participate in a CAI session and their overall enjoyment throughout the session. As raised previously, we recommend that handlers assess their dog's consent to participate at multiple points throughout a CAI session; as is the case with human participants, therapy dog consent might wax and wane. In this way, to optimize welfare and enjoyment in CAIs, therapy dog consent must be conceptualized as dynamically unfolding in real time and within a lively context, thus requiring ongoing assessment throughout the session. Further, to respect the therapy dog's agency in a CAI session, handlers can take concrete action by immediately ending a session, taking a short break, changing the setting, or identifying and removing the causes of stress before resuming a session (Ameli et al., 2023).

EMOTIONAL CONTAGION IN DOG-HANDLER TEAMS

The owner/handler and dog are evaluated and approved to participate together as a dyad in CAI programs. The unique bond and communication between them contribute to the safe practice of CAI and attention to canine welfare.

(Barker & Gee, 2021, p. 7)

In the above quotation, the handler and therapy dog form a *dyad* or *team* to ensure the safe practice of CAI for both humans and canines. Barker and Gee (2021) cite this conceptualization as critical to the successful implementation of the *Dogs on Call Program* which was established in the Center for Human-Animal Interaction at Virginia Commonwealth University School of Medicine in 2001. As discussed in Chapter 3, in humans, the process of emotional contagion is well documented and shown to unfold in dynamic applied settings including classrooms between teachers and students (e.g., elevated teacher stress influenced students' cortisol levels; Oberle & Schonert-Reichl, 2016), and healthcare settings between healthcare providers and clients (e.g., nurses absorbed their patient's joy and anger; Petitta et al., 2016). Recent research highlights the unique bond and emotional communication patterns shared between humans and dogs, and that dogs are attuned to their owners'/handlers' emotional states (Müller et al., 2015). For instance, studies have shown that emotional contagion (or emotional state matching) between dogs and their owners/handlers can occur when dogs show physiologic and behavioural attuning to human signs of distress (Custance & Mayer, 2012; Yong & Ruffman, 2014). In one study, both humans and dogs showed heightened alertness and increased cortisol levels from baseline only after listening to the sounds of human infants crying (Yong & Ruffman, 2014). In another study, dogs showed what appeared like empathically motivated prosocial helping to humans in need (Sanford et al., 2018).

In the context of CAIs, a therapy dog might reflect their handler's positive or negative emotional state, and handlers might also reflect their dog's feelings of enjoyment, anxiety, or discomfort. Such emotional and behavioural attuning to their owners/handlers could serve to strengthen the bond between the therapy dog and their handler and contribute to the overall level of stress or enjoyment experienced by the dyad within a CAI session. As described in Chapter 3, research by Silas and colleagues (2019) found that 25% of the handlers in their sample of 40 dog-handler teams who reported elevated stress also had dogs characterized by heightened stress. In this case, it is possible that the handlers' emotional state was implicitly transmitted to their therapy dogs. We reiterate here that clients can be best supported when the therapy dog-handler team is relaxed, and the team's welfare has been carefully considered (Figure 5.5).

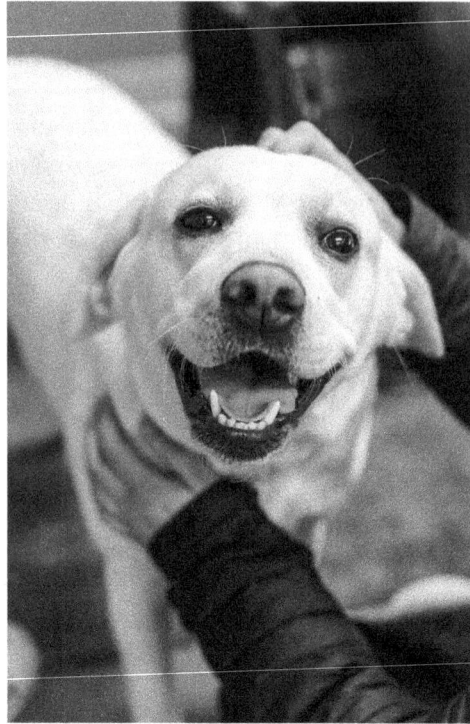

Figure 5.5 Therapy dog Cali demonstrates her contentment as she smiles with an open mouth and bright eyes while being gently stroked behind her ears and on her shoulder
Source: Madisyn Szypula and F. L. L. Green Photography; used with permission

BEST PRACTICES IN OPTIMIZING THERAPY DOG-HANDLER TEAM WELFARE AND ENJOYMENT IN CAIS

As we have discussed so far, several factors and challenges can contribute to therapy dog and handler stress and undermine welfare and enjoyment while participating in CAIs. Drawing on our own and others' published research on developing and implementing both in person (Bailey, 2023; Baird et al., 2022; Binfet et al., 2022a; 2022b; 2018; 2017; Kivlen et al., 2022; Pendry et al., 2018; Pendry & Vandagriff, 2019; Wood et al., 2018) and virtual (Binfet et al., 2022a; Dell et al., 2021; Steel, 2023; Tardif-Williams et al., 2023) CAIs to support university students' well-being, we offer the following recommendations for best practices in optimizing therapy dog-handler welfare and

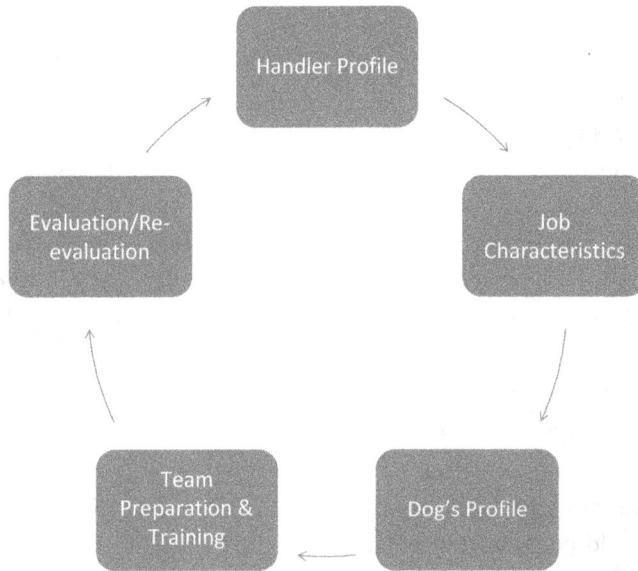

Figure 5.6 An illustration of dog-handler engagement
Source: Winkle et al., 2020; used with permission from *Animals*

enjoyment in CAIs. We also draw on a framework put forward by Winkle and colleagues (2020) in the context of animal-assisted therapy, and we note that some of these recommendations are preparatory, whereas others are to be executed continuously; some highlight aspects the handler's and dog's preferences and energy levels; and still others highlight dynamic aspects of the environment in which CAIs unfold (see Figure 5.6).

Winkle and colleagues (2020) note that the core tenets of biomedical practice (i.e., boundaries of competence, altruism, prudence) should also extend to therapy dogs involved in CAIs and note that this "means doing right by the dog even when it does not serve the client" (p. 6). These authors suggest that in addition to the basic tenets of biomedical practice, therapy dog handlers should have a working knowledge and application of animal learning theory, interspecies communication, and humane training techniques. Research, however, shows that animal-assisted programs (including CAIs) vary widely in terms of processes for handler and dog team preparation, training, and evaluation (Serpell et al., 2020). Thus, to optimize welfare in CAIs, we highly recommend that therapy dog-handler teams take part in advance preparation and training (Winkle et al., 2020). This advance preparation and training should focus on ensuring a good match – or *goodness of fit* – between therapy dog and handler energy levels and preferences for type and number of clients and session activities. Also, in keeping with research on the importance of emotional contagion within therapy dog-handler teams, we encourage program personnel to develop protocols to support handlers in doing an initial health check on their dog's emotional and physical welfare prior to the start of each CAI session; this is an important first step in optimizing therapy dog welfare within CAIs. Similarly, we encourage handlers to engage in emotional self-reflection before participating in each session. Dogs whose handlers are feeling anxious or tense might also show signs of physiologic and behavioural distress – through a process of emotional state matching. In this case, the welfare of the therapy dog-handler team would be compromised as would their ability to support clients in CAIs. Handlers should be encouraged and afforded the flexibility from booking institutions, program personnel, and visiting clients to cancel their participation in a session if either they or their dog is not feeling optimally well and/or ready to participate in a CAI session. As discussed in Chapter 3, optimizing the welfare of dog-handler teams is the shared responsibility of all the agents involved in the organization, delivery, and oversight of CAIs.

Therapy dog welfare and enjoyment must also be monitored continuously during a CAI session. In this regard, some of the practical factors to consider involve the environment in which CAIs unfold such as offering sufficient spacing (attending to room density), making water and comfort blankets available, offering several toilet breaks if needed. We also consider if dogs are comfortable being positioned in a particular area or station of the room. In this regard, we consider the dog's room temperature preferences and preference for proximity to neighbouring dogs. For instance, younger and less experienced dogs might prefer to have their own quieter station in the room, and some dogs also feel uncomfortable being positioned nearby an unfamiliar dog. We also consider whether a station offers lower or higher stimulation or greater flow through traffic of clients, and we position dogs according to their preferences. For instance, some dogs enjoy interacting with high-energy clients who engage in more direct physical touching such as younger children, whereas other dogs enjoy interacting with less energetic clients who engage in less physical contact (perhaps only ambiently) such as people receiving medical care. Some of these contingencies are especially relevant when delivering CAIs to larger groups of clients, as compared to when CAIs are delivered in one-on-one contexts. However, each of these contingencies is important to consider when optimizing therapy dog-handler team welfare enjoyment in CAIs. Other factors to consider involve the duration of individual sessions, the number of sessions per week in which animal-handler teams participate, the number of new environments animals are required to adapt to, and the number and behaviour of clients/visitors supported. Regarding session length, while there is variation in the duration of individual sessions across CAI contexts, the trend in CAI research is to use abbreviated sessions lasting approximately 15–20 minutes (for a review, see Binfet & Hartwig, 2020). However, we recognize that in practice CAIs often vary in duration and consideration should be given to the dog's preference for the length of individual sessions and total number of sessions per week. Also, clients should observe rules pertaining to cleanliness and hygiene, consent-to-pet, and feeding food and treats to therapy dogs. These are all factors that can individually and collectively compromise therapy animal welfare, and that require continual monitoring throughout CAIs.

Another factor to consider in optimizing therapy dog-handler team welfare is the availability of human support such as program personnel to assist and support. Here, some key questions are: Is there a designated human responsible for monitoring and verifying therapy dog welfare during CAIs? Does the designated monitor have sufficient training and experience in monitoring and verifying animal welfare? Does the designated monitor have experience with recognizing breed-specific nuances in dog's emotional and behavioural communication patterns? Is the designated monitor sufficiently familiar with the dog that is to be included as part of the CAI? Are they the most appropriate person to assign to monitor the welfare of a particular dog? Is there a good, designated dog welfare monitor-to-dog ratio? As noted previously, we position handlers as key advocates for their therapy dogs and overseers ensuring the successful implementation of welfare measures to support their dog's participation and welfare during CAIs. Handlers are most familiar with their dog's baseline stress levels and nuanced emotional and behavioural communication patterns; in this way, welfare checks are perhaps easier to conduct and more sensitive.

It is also important to develop a contingency protocol in the event of an unusual, but potentially stressful event. For instance, dogs (and handlers) can become stressed by a loud sounding fire drill and the loud sound and fast-paced, frantic movements that accompany such an event. In this regard, some questions to consider include: Is there an adequate protocol in place to keep therapy dog handler teams physically safe during sessions? Does everyone know the evacuation spot? Does the session resume or conclude after such an event? Is there a protocol to calm stressed therapy dog-handler teams after such an event or prior to resuming a session – as dogs could experience stress after such an event and upon re-entering the space on future occasions?

Promisingly, we have outlined several strategies to optimize the welfare and enjoyment of the therapy dog-handler team within the context of CAIs. Importantly, we also support Winkle and colleagues' (2020) best practices recommendation that therapy dog-handler teams undergo regular (perhaps annual) evaluations to ensure program implementation fidelity and to optimize both therapy dog and handler welfare. See Table 5.3 for a *Welfare Checklist: Considerations in Optimizing Welfare for Therapy Dog-Handler Teams*.

Table 5.3 Welfare Checklist: Considerations in Optimizing Welfare for Therapy Dog-Handler Teams

---

- Has the therapy dog-handler team undergone screening to determine suitability for the type of participation in question? (i.e., Has the therapy dog's potential to participate in a CAI session been assessed?)
- Has the therapy dog-handler team engaged in advance training and practice or simulation sessions to determine suitability for the type of participation in question? (i.e., Does the therapy dog-handler team feel prepared to engage with the clients and environment comfortably and optimally?)
- Has the handler been provided training/practice/education regarding how to optimally interact with the client(s)?

Table 5.3 (Cont.)

- Has the space been prepared for the team? (i.e., swept and cleaned, verified for sharp objects, dropped food and medication, etc.)
- Have the clients been provided education/instruction on how to optimally interact with the therapy dog?
- Has the handler conducted a health check on their dog's emotional and physical welfare and readiness to participate in the session?
- Has the handler engaged in emotional self-reflection to confirm readiness to participate in the session?
- Is the room temperature being monitored to prevent the therapy dog from overheating?
- Are water and comfort blankets available before, during, and after the session?
- Are toilet breaks offered before, during, and after the session?
- Have time-out breaks been scheduled as part of each session?
- Are cleanliness and hygiene rules being observed by all participants?
- Are rules about giving the dog food and treats being observed by all participants?
- Is there sufficient spacing to prevent overcrowding?
- Is the session length and number of clients appropriate to the dog's and handler's preferences?
- Is the duration of the intervention and the number of interventions per day in accordance with recommended best practices?
- Are the planned session activities appropriate to the dog's preferences for human contact and energy levels?
- Are there program personnel present to assist and support the therapy dog-handler team?
- Have efforts been made to obtain consent from the therapy dog?
- Does the interaction encourage the therapy dog to demonstrate natural behaviours?
- Is the therapy dog able to escape or retreat from clients or is the therapy dog surrounded? Can the therapy dog walk away?
- Is the therapy dog's agency respected? Is the therapy dog determining participation and able to voluntarily cease to participate?
- Is there a designated human responsible for monitoring and verifying therapy dog welfare during CAIs? If not, how will the handler monitor welfare whilst concurrently overseeing the CAI session?
- Does the designated monitor have sufficient training and experience in monitoring and verifying animal welfare? Does the designated monitor have experience with recognizing breed-specific nuances in dog's emotional and behavioural communication patterns? Is the designated monitor sufficiently familiar with the dog that is to be included as part of the CAI? Are they the most appropriate person to assign to monitor the welfare of a particular dog?

(continued)

Table 5.3 (Cont.)

- Has an optimal welfare monitor-to-dog ratio been established?
- Have barriers or deterrents to reporting adverse effects been acknowledged/recognized? (i.e., reflecting poorly on the agency)
-
- Is there an adequate protocol in place in the event of an unusual, but potentially stressful event (e.g., fire drill) to keep therapy dog-handler teams physically safe during sessions? Does everyone know the evacuation spot? Does the session resume or conclude after such an event? Is there a protocol to calm stressed therapy dog-handler teams after such an event or prior to resuming a session – as dogs could experience stress after such an event and upon re-entering the space on future occasions?
- Is there a plan in place for therapy dog-handler teams to undergo regular (perhaps annual) evaluations to ensure program implementation fidelity and to optimize both therapy dog and handler welfare?

CONCLUSION

Interest in optimizing therapy dog welfare in the context of CAIs has burgeoned over the past decade, and CAI scholars and practitioners share a common understanding that supporting clients effectively depends on the welfare of the therapy dog-handler team. Building upon the foundational information shared thus far in our book, in this chapter, we discussed how, despite best intentions, a therapy dog's welfare may be compromised within a CAI session. We considered how dynamic applied contexts present a whole host of potential threats to the welfare of both the therapy dog and handler. As part of this chapter, we included an ethogram of indicators or signs of canine stress, and we discussed factors potentially undermining a dog-handler team's welfare and ability to support human clients. We also discussed variables and conditions that help optimize the welfare of dog-handler teams. This included a discussion of the importance of attending to therapy dog welfare, enjoyment, and agency in CAIs. We also considered the handler's role as an educator and advocate, how handlers can reduce risk to therapy dog welfare by educating visiting clients, how to implement the concept of therapy dog consent, and the role of emotional contagion in dog-handler teams. Last, as part of this chapter, we provided readers with recommendations for best practices and offered a checklist supporting and guiding readers in optimizing welfare for both therapy dogs and handlers in the context of CAIs. We now turn to a discussion of the varied contexts in which CAIs unfold and some of the real-time challenges that handlers can face when assessing and managing their therapy dog's stress.

REFERENCES

Ameli, K., Braun, T. F., & Krämer, S. (2023). Animal-assisted interventions and animal welfare—an exploratory survey in Germany. *Animals*, 13(8), 1324. https://doi.org/10.3390/ani13081324

Bailey, K. (2023). A scoping review of campus-based animal-assisted interactions programs for college student mental health. *People and Animals: The International Journal of Research and Practice*, 6(1), 1–27. https://doi.org/10.62845/iqjlqog

Baird, R., Grové, C., & Berger, E. (2022). The impact of therapy dogs on the social and emotional wellbeing of students: A systematic review. *Educational and Developmental Psychologist*, 39(2), 180–208. https://doi.org/10.1080/20590776.2022.2049444

Barker, S. B., & Gee, N. R. (2021). Canine-assisted interventions in hospitals: Best practices for maximizing human and canine safety. *Frontiers in Veterinary Science*, 8, 1–12. https://doi.org/10.3389/fvets.2021.615730

Binfet, J.-T., Green, F. L., & Draper, Z. A. (2022a). The importance of client–canine contact in canine-assisted interventions: A randomized controlled trial. *Anthrozoös*, 35(1), 1–22. https://doi.org/10.1080/08927936.2021.1944558

Binfet, J.-T., & Hartwig, E. K. (2020). *Canine-assisted interventions: A comprehensive guide to credentialing therapy dog teams*. Routledge.

Custance, D., & Mayer, J. (2012). Empathic-like responding by domestic dogs (canis familiaris) to distress in humans: An exploratory study. *Animal Cognition*, 15(5), 851–859. https://doi.org/10.1007/s10071-012-0510-1

Dell, C., Williamson, L., McKenzie, H., Carey, B., Cruz, M., Gibson, M., & Pavelich, A. (2021). A commentary about lessons learned: Transitioning a therapy dog program online during the COVID-19 pandemic. *Animals*, 11(3), 914. https://doi.org/10.3390/ani11030914

Enders-Slegers, M.-J., & Hediger, K. (2019). Pet ownership and human–animal interaction in an aging population: Rewards and challenges. *Anthrozoös*, 32(2), 255–265. https://doi.org/10.1080/08927936.2019.1569907

Fatjó, J., Bown, J., & Calvo, P. (2021). Stress in therapy animals. In J. M. Peralta & A. Fine (Eds.), *The welfare of animals in animal-assisted interventions: Foundations and best practice methods* (pp. 91–121). Springer.

Gee, N. R. (2023). Animals in education. *The Routledge International Handbook of Human-Animal Interactions and Anthrozoology* (1st ed., pp. 509–521). https://doi.org/10.4324/9781032153346-35

Glenk, L. (2017). Current perspectives on therapy dog welfare in animal-assisted interventions. *Animals*, 7(12), 7. https://doi.org/10.3390/ani7020007

Glenk, L. M., & Foltin, S. (2021). Therapy dog welfare revisited: A review of the literature. *Veterinary Sciences*, 8(10), 226. https://doi.org/10.3390/vetsci8100226

Hatch, A. (2007). The view from all fours: A look at an animal-assisted activity program from the animals' perspective. *Anthrozoös*, 20(1), 37–50. https://doi.org/10.2752/089279307780216632

Haubenhofer, D. K., & Kirchengast, S. (2006). Physiological arousal for companion dogs working with their owners in animal-assisted activities and animal-assisted therapy. *Journal of Applied Animal Welfare Science*, 9(2), 165–172. https://doi.org/10.1207/s15327604jaws0902_5

Horowitz, A. (2021). Considering the "dog" in dog–human interaction. *Frontiers in Veterinary Science*, 8, 1–5. https://doi.org/10.3389/fvets.2021.642821

Iannuzzi, D., & Rowan, A. N. (1991). Ethical issues in animal-assisted therapy programs. *Anthrozoös*, 4(3), 154–163. https://doi.org/10.2752/089279391787057116

Iqbal, U., Williams, J. M., & Knoll, M. (2023). An evaluation of a canine welfare education intervention for primary school children. *Anthrozoös*, 37(2), 303–322. https://doi.org/10.1080/08927936.2023.2268978

Jegatheesan, B., Beetz, A., Ormerod, E., Johnson, R., Fine, A. H., Yamazaki, K., Dudzik, C., Garcia, R. M., Winkle, M., & Choi, G. (2019). The IAHAIO definitions for animal assisted intervention and guidelines for wellness of animals involved in AAI. In A. H. Fine (Ed.), *Handbook on animal-assisted therapy* (5th ed., pp. 500–501). Elsevier Academic Press.

King, C., Watters, J., & Mungre, S. (2011). Effect of a time-out session with working animal-assisted therapy dogs. *Journal of Veterinary Behavior*, 6(4), 232–238. https://doi.org/10.1016/j.jveb.2011.01.007

Kivlen, C., Winston, K., Mills, D., DiZazzo-Miller, R., Davenport, R., & Binfet, J.-T. (2022). Canine-assisted intervention effects on the well-being of health science graduate students: A randomized controlled trial. *The American Journal of Occupational Therapy*, 76(6), 1–8. https://doi.org/10.5014/ajot.2022.049508

Mariti, C., Gazzano, A., Moore, J. L., Baragli, P., Chelli, L., & Sighieri, C. (2012). Perception of dogs' stress by their owners. *Journal of Veterinary Behavior*, 7(4), 213–219. https://doi.org/10.1016/j.jveb.2011.09.004

McCullough, A., Jenkins, M. A., Ruehrdanz, A., Gilmer, M. J., Olson, J., Pawar, A., Holley, L., Sierra-Rivera, S., Linder, D. E., Pichette, D., Grossman, N. J., Hellman, C., Guérin, N. A., & O'Haire, M. E. (2018). Physiological and behavioral effects of animal-assisted interventions on therapy dogs in pediatric oncology settings. *Applied Animal Behaviour Science*, 200, 86–95. https://doi.org/10.1016/j.applanim.2017.11.014

Meints, K., Brelsford, V., & De Keuster, T. (2018). Teaching children and parents to understand dog signaling. *Frontiers in Veterinary Science*, 5, 1–14. https://doi.org/10.3389/fvets.2018.00257

Mellor, D. (2016). Updating animal welfare thinking: Moving beyond the "five freedoms" towards "A life worth living." *Animals*, 6(3), 21. https://doi.org/10.3390/ani6030021

Mignot, A., de Luca, K., Servais, V., & Leboucher, G. (2022). Handlers' representations on therapy dogs' welfare. *Animals*, 12(5), 580. https://doi.org/10.3390/ani12050580

Müller, C. A., Schmitt, K., Barber, A. L. A., & Huber, L. (2015). Dogs can discriminate emotional expressions of human faces. *Current Biology*, 25(5), 601–605. https://doi.org/10.1016/j.cub.2014.12.055

Ng, Z. (2021). Strategies to assessing and enhancing animal welfare in animal-assisted interventions. In J. M. Peralta & A. Fine (Eds.), *The welfare of animals in animal-assisted interventions: Foundations and best practice methods* (pp. 123–154). Springer.

Ng, Z., Albright, J., Fine, A. H., & Peralta, J. (2015). Our ethical and moral responsibility: Ensuring the welfare of therapy animals. In Aubrey H. Fine (Ed.), *Handbook on animal-assisted therapy: Foundations and guidelines for animal-assisted interventions* (4th ed., pp. 91–101). Elsevier/Academic Press.

Ng, Z., & Fine, A. H. (2021). A trajectory approach to supporting therapy animal welfare in retirement and beyond. In J. M. Peralta & A. Fine (Eds.), *The welfare of animals in animal-assisted interventions: Foundations and best practice methods* (pp. 243–263). Springer.

Novack, L. I., Schnell-Peskin, L., Feuerbacher, E., & Fernandez, E. J. (2023). The science and social validity of companion animal welfare: Functionally defined parameters in a multidisciplinary field. *Animals*, 13(11), 1850. https://doi.org/10.3390/ani13111850

Oberle, E., & Schonert-Reichl, K. A. (2016). Stress contagion in the classroom? The link between classroom teacher burnout and morning cortisol in elementary school students. *Social Science & Medicine*, 159, 30–37. https://doi.org/10.1016/j.socscimed.2016.04.031

Overall, K. L. (2013). *Manual of clinical behavioral medicine for dogs and cats.* Elsevier.

Pendry, P., Carr, A. M., Roeter, S. M., & Vandagriff, J. L. (2018). Experimental trial demonstrates effects of animal-assisted stress prevention program on college students' positive and negative emotion. *Human-Animal Interaction Bulletin*, 6(1), 81–97. https://doi.org/10.1079/hai.2018.0004

Pendry, P., & Vandagriff, J. L. (2019). Animal visitation program (AVP) reduces cortisol levels of university students: A randomized controlled trial. *AERA Open*, 5(2), 1–12. https://doi.org/10.1177/2332858419852592

Peralta, J. M., & Fine, A. H. (2021). The welfarist and the psychologist: Finding common ground in our interactions with therapy animals. In J. M. Peralta & A. Fine (Eds.), *The welfare of animals in animal-assisted interventions: Foundations and best practice methods* (pp. 265–284). Springer.

Peralta, J. M., & Fine, A. H. (2021). *The welfare of animals in animal-assisted interventions: Foundations and best practice methods.* Springer.

Petitta, L., Jiang, L., & Härtel, C. E. J. (2016). Emotional contagion and burnout among nurses and doctors: Do joy and anger from different sources of stakeholders matter?. *Stress and Health*, 33(4), 358–369. https://doi.org/10.1002/smi.2724

Provoost, L. (2021). Behavior and training for optimal welfare in therapy settings. In J. M. Peralta & A. Fine (Eds.), *The welfare of animals in animal-assisted interventions: Foundations and best practice methods* (pp. 59–90). Springer.

Sanford, E. M., Burt, E. R., & Meyers-Manor, J. E. (2018). Timmy's in the well: Empathy and prosocial helping in dogs. *Learning & Behavior, 46*(4), 374–386. https://doi.org/10.3758/s13420-018-0332-3

Sarrafchi, A., David-Steel, M., Pearce, S. D., de Zwaan, N., & Merkies, K. (2022). Effect of human-dog interaction on therapy dog stress during an on-campus student stress buster event. *Applied Animal Behaviour Science, 253*, 105659. https://doi.org/10.1016/j.applanim.2022.105659

Serpell, J. A., Kruger, K. A., Freeman, L. M., Griffin, J. A., & Ng, Z. Y. (2020). Current standards and practices within the therapy dog industry: Results of a representative survey of United States therapy dog organizations. *Frontiers in Veterinary Science, 7*, 1–12. https://doi.org/10.3389/fvets.2020.00035

Shepherd, K. (2002). Development of behavior, social behavior and communication in dogs. In D. F. Horwitz & D. S. Mills (Eds.), *BSAVA manual of canine and feline behaviour medicine* (pp. 8–20). British Small Animal Veterinary Association.

Silas, H. J., Binfet, J.-T., & Ford, A. T. (2019). Therapeutic for all? Observational assessments of therapy canine stress in an on-campus stress-reduction program. *Journal of Veterinary Behavior, 32*, 6–13. https://doi.org/10.1016/j.jveb.2019.03.009

Spinka, M. (2019). Animal agency, animal awareness and animal welfare. *Animal Welfare, 28*(1), 11–20. https://doi.org/10.7120/09627286.28.1.011

Steel, J. (2023). Reading to dogs in schools: A controlled feasibility study of an online reading to dogs intervention. *International Journal of Educational Research, 117*, 102117. https://doi.org/10.1016/j.ijer.2022.102117

Tardif-Williams, C. Y., & Binfet, J.-T. (2023). Virtual human-animal interactions. *Routledge*. https://doi.org/10.4324/9781003327868

Townsend, L., & Gee, N. R. (2021). Recognizing and mitigating canine stress during animal assisted interventions. *Veterinary Sciences, 8*(11), 254. https://doi.org/10.3390/vetsci8110254

Uccheddu, S., Albertini, M., Pierantoni, L., Fantino, S., & Pirrone, F. (2018). Assessing behavior and stress in two dogs during sessions of a reading-to-a-dog program for children with pervasive developmental disorders. *Dog Behavior, 4*, 1–12.

VanFleet, R. (2014). *What it means to be humane in animal-assisted interventions*. Academia. edu. https://www.academia.edu/33218547/What_It_Means_to_Be_Humane_in_Animal_Assisted_Interventions

Winkle, M., & Johnson Binder, A. (2024). The importance of animal welfare in animal-assisted services. *Animal Behaviour and Welfare Cases*, 1–4. https://doi.org/10.1079/abwcases.2024.0003

Winkle, M., Johnson, A., & Mills, D. (2020). Dog welfare, well-being and behavior: Considerations for selection, evaluation and suitability for animal-assisted therapy. *Animals, 10*(11), 2188. https://doi.org/10.3390/ani10112188

Wood, E., Ohlsen, S., Thompson, J., Hulin, J., & Knowles, L. (2018). The feasibility of brief dog-assisted therapy on university students stress levels: The paws study. *Journal of Mental Health*, 27(3), 263–268. https://doi.org/10.1080/09638237.2017.1385737

Yong, M. H., & Ruffman, T. (2014). Emotional contagion: Dogs and humans show a similar physiological response to human infant crying. *Behavioural Processes*, 108, 155–165. https://doi.org/10.1016/j.beproc.2014.10.006

Six

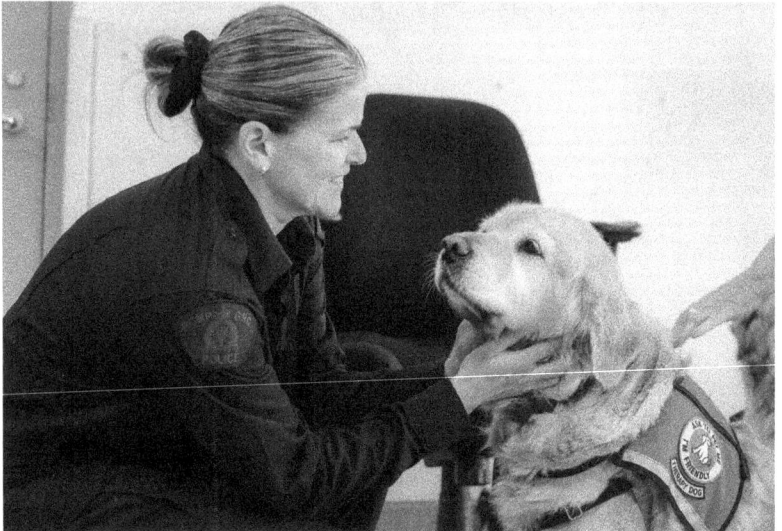

Figure 6.1 During a session within the detachment, a police member cups the face of therapy dog Dash, a Golden Retriever

Source: Photo credit: F. L. L. Green Photography; used with permission

DOI: 10.4324/9781032639284-6

SCENARIO

Therapy Dogs and Youth Involved in the Criminal Justice System Making Connections and Sharing Hope

Arya is a youth services officer working for a medium-sized detention centre which houses incarcerated youth between the ages of 12 and 17 years. Arya's job involves organizing rehabilitation programs and activities for diverse youth with the goal of steering them away from engaging in further criminal acts. Being an avid dog lover who lives with two large companion dogs, Arya is keen to launch a program that would bring together therapy dogs and youth who are incarcerated. He has read about the growing popularity of such programs, which highlight the special and mutually rewarding bonds that can develop between dogs and incarcerated youth. Arya wonders: Where do I start? How can I develop a safe and successful therapy dog program? Arya wants to ensure the safety of both the dog-handler team and the incarcerated youth under his care; he proceeds with caution, despite his enthusiasm for the project. Arya knows that some of the youth have trouble with social connections and empathy, which can sometimes lead to unpredictable emotional and behavioural outbursts. Some of them are known to openly express anger and behave aggressively. Arya is passionate about dogs and wants his therapy dog program to succeed for both the dogs and the incarcerated youth; thus, he reaches out to human-animal interaction (HAI) researchers at a nearby university to suggest best practices for optimizing the welfare of the dog-handler team and the youth involved (Figure 6.1).

QUESTIONS FOR REFLECTION AND DISCUSSION

1. What are the unique considerations for therapy dog-handler teams working across specialized settings and with specialized clients?

2. To optimize therapy dog welfare in specialized settings and with specialized clients, what conditions should be in place for therapy dogs?

3. Should a handler be required to receive training before engaging therapy dogs in their practice across different settings and with different populations such as in a detention centre for youth involved in the criminal justice system? Should a handler collect information about clients' past experiences with therapy dogs (animals)?

4. Should professionals such as Arya, a youth services worker, be required to receive training prior to introducing incarcerated youth to a therapy dog? What guidance should specialized clients such as youth involved in the criminal justice system receive in advance of meeting a dog-handler team?

5. How should therapy dog sessions be structured within specialized settings involving diverse clients such as a correctional facility for youth involved in the criminal justice system? Where should sessions unfold and how much supervision should they involve? How long should sessions last?

ILLUSTRATION OF THE VARIABILITY IN CONTEXTS AND CLIENTS

Health and human service professionals uphold an oath to "Do No Harm" (and beyond that, doing right by the dog) and that tenet must extend to the dogs who are working in a professional capacity with the clinician.

(Winkle et al., 2020, p. 11)

As the field of HAIs broadens and extends its reach, so too do we see CAIs implemented in a variety of new contexts in support of the well-being of diverse clients. The rapid growth in CAIs in applied, dynamic settings raises unique concerns for therapy dog welfare (Binfet & Hartwig, 2020; Bremhorst & Mills, 2021). The scenario at the outset of this chapter highlights the challenging and dynamic context that can emerge when a dog-handler team visits a facility for youth involved in the criminal justice system. In Chapter 5, we touched upon how CAIs occur in diverse settings and involve challenging and dynamic interactions among various agents, including the dog-handler therapy team, the client, and support personnel (e.g., teacher, child advocate, clinician, youth justice worker). We also discussed how these varied contexts and clients are replete with several unknown, unpredictable, and ever-changing variables, thus raising unique considerations for dog-handler welfare. In this chapter, we take a closer look at some of the settings that feature CAIs and the specialized populations they serve and discuss some of the associated welfare considerations. We also address Arya's question about best practices for optimizing therapy dog-handler team welfare in highly specialized contexts such as a detention centre for youth involved in the criminal justice system. In the sections that follow, we consider dog-handler welfare within educational settings, medical settings, prison and correctional facilities, virtual contexts, and specialized settings involving specialized populations (e.g., airports, crisis response settings, workplace and recreational settings, funeral homes, homeless shelters, long-term care facilities, police detachments and military bases, and public libraries).

ENSURING DOG-HANDLER TEAM WELFARE IN EDUCATIONAL SETTINGS

Increasingly, we see therapy dogs being integrated into educational settings ranging from elementary to post-secondary levels to support student reading, learning, and social-emotional competencies (for reviews, see Baird et al., 2023; Binfet & Hartwig, 2020; Grové et al., 2021; Hall et al., 2017; Reilly et al., 2020; Renck Jalongo & Petro, 2018; Sandt, 2020; Tardif-Williams & Binfet, 2023; Townsend & Gee, 2021). Frequently, therapy dogs are included as part of programs to support student reading skills as dogs foster a welcoming and non-threatening environment in which to practice reading. Such therapy dog reading programs often take place within classrooms (e.g., Kirnan et al., 2016), after-school settings or libraries (e.g., Rousseau & Tardif-Williams, 2019), and virtual contexts (Steel, 2023). Also, school- and campus-based therapy dogs are becoming increasingly popular adjuncts in student-directed learning and wellness efforts (Bailey, 2023; Baird et al., 2022; Barker et al., 2016; Binfet, 2017; Binfet et al., 2018; Crossman et al., 2015; Kivlen et al., 2022; Pendry et al., 2018; Pendry & Vandagriff, 2019; Wood et al., 2018). However, there are important welfare considerations when students interact with therapy dogs, which are often unaddressed in the literature on the safe and successful implementation of CAIs within educational settings (Fine, 2019; Gee & Fine, 2019).

In a qualitative study conducted by Baird and colleagues (2023), school personnel raised concerns about the welfare and safety risks for both students and therapy dogs when they interact. Practically, some student welfare concerns related to interactions with therapy dogs included allergies, health conditions, and individuals with a fear of dogs (Baird et al., 2023; Grové et al., 2021). In turn, concerns have also been raised regarding therapy dog welfare in educational contexts such overstimulation, overcrowding, and overwork (Glenk, 2017; Meints et al., 2018). One welfare concern is that therapy dogs might be overstimulated when interacting with younger children. For instance, one study found that therapy dogs' stress-associated behaviours increased during sessions with young children (aged less than 12 years) as compared to more senior people, which might be because younger children offer more stimulating and unpredictable interactions as compared to older people (Marinelli et al., 2009). Another welfare concern is that therapy dogs might experience overcrowding when CAIs are held in more confined spaces (e.g., Baird et al., 2023; King et al., 2011; Meints et al., 2018), especially when they are simultaneously approached by several enthusiastic students. Therapy dogs might also experience overworking when CAI sessions last longer than is optimal and involve many students (e.g., Baird et al., 2022). Further, Townsend and Gee (2021) note that certain physical aspects of educational settings can compromise the welfare of therapy dogs (see Figure 6.2). These include slippery floors; excessively hot or cold room or floor/pavement temperatures; loud, unfamiliar, or unexpected noises (e.g., ringing school bell, voices over intercom speaker); the presence of other dogs or classroom animals; confined spaces; and the lack of options for the dog to move away from people or leave the room (Table 6.1).

Further, Townsend and Gee (2021) highlight several practical human-related aspects specific to dynamic and busy educational environments that can potentially impact the welfare of the therapy dog. These include having multiple people in the room, including children and youth of various developmental ages and abilities; students' loud and random vocalizations and behaviours; simultaneous and competing attempts from students to interact with the therapy dog; and lack of knowledge on how to safely approach and touch the therapy dog, potentially leading some children to handle a therapy

Table 6.1 Mitigation Strategies

Environmental Characteristics	Canine Stressors	Handler Contingencies	Mitigation Strategies
• Nursing home visitation • Hospital visitation • Employee wellness event • University studies stress relief	• Crowds • High noise level • Unfamiliar sounds • Multiple people touching dog • No pathway for animal to disengage or leave • Slick floors • Hot weather • Hot pavement • Multiple dogs present	• High activity level • Heightened attentional demands • Crowd control • Lengthy/ indeterminate interaction time • Desire to make patients/ visitors feel better • Pressure to interact/ entertain • Constant need to watch the clock	• Thorough handler training in recognizing early signs of canine stress • Frequent breaks to allow "escape" • People on hand for crowd control and observation of dog • Scheduling multiple dogs for shorter time frames and rotate them into and out of interactions • Temperature mitigation techniques such as ice cubes or water • Setting up interaction for success, i.e., treats to motivate the dog to interact • Set timer to check in with the dog/ give them a break • Monitor how the dog does at home after interaction; adjust future visits accordingly

Source: Townsend & Gee., 2021; used with permission from *Veterinary Sciences*

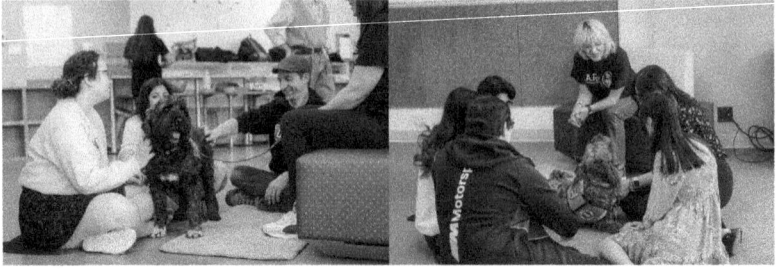

Figure 6.2 The staged photo on the right shows overcrowding with several students trying to simultaneously touch a therapy dog who has no clear exit path, whereas the image on the left shows only two students touching a content and smiling therapy dog who has a clear exit path.
Source: F. L. L. Green Photography; used with permission

dog roughly (e.g., pulling ears or tail, hugging, touching or blowing in sensitive areas) and making loud noises that could startle the dog.

Further, educational contexts often include groups of diverse learners of varying ages and competencies including, but not limited to, learners who have disabilities (e.g., autism, attention-deficit hyperactivity disorder), mental health challenges (e.g., post-traumatic stress disorder, aggression, anxiety, depression), behavioural challenges (e.g., aggression, impulsivity), and people within diverse sociodemographic communities (e.g., Indigenous, individuals experiencing homelessness/marginalized, Black, Indigenous, and People of Color, and Two-Spirit, lesbian, gay, bisexual, transgender, queer, intersex, and additional people who identify as part of sexual and gender diverse communities). Student diversity must be considered when designing CAIs to optimize therapy dog welfare in complex and fast-paced educational contexts (Gee et al., 2017; Townsend & Gee, 2021). Dynamic and busy educational settings involving diverse students might raise unique welfare challenges for therapy dog-handler teams. For instance, it is possible that students who have intellectual or developmental disabilities (e.g., attention-deficit hyperactivity disorder, autism spectrum disorder) might interact in a way that a therapy dog finds uncomfortable or overwhelming (i.e., talk too loudly into the dog's ear; make loud and random vocalizations; hug the dog too closely, tightly, or for too long; restrict the dog's bid to move away). Students who experience heightened anxiety which often characterizes learners in the post-secondary context who deal with many competing stressors or students who experience post-traumatic stress disorder due to past trauma might transmit their anxiety or emotional discomfort onto therapy dogs who might be ill-equipped to manage intense emotions. Other aspects of student diversity such as impulsivity and aggressive behavioural tendencies might also compromise therapy dog welfare. Without warning, a child might quickly pull on a dog's tail or ears. Handlers and school personnel should prepare for such contingencies in advance of a CAI session. Students will also vary in terms of their past experiences with diverse animals (e.g., farm, companion, wild) which might shape their knowledge about, attitudes towards, and treatment of animals. For instance, students might respond fearfully towards a dog due to a past encounter that was perceived as traumatic (e.g., being harmed by a dog). The design and implementation of CAIs should consider students' past animal-related experiences and offer some advance education about how to interact with therapy dogs optimally and respectfully (Baird et al., 2023; Gee et al., 2017; Townsend & Gee, 2021).

SCREENING PROTOCOLS AND TRAINING FOR THERAPY DOG-HANDLER TEAM

In qualitative research conducted by Baird and colleagues (2023) on the successful implementation of CAIs, school personnel cited the importance of client education to outline expectations and guidelines for how students should optimally interact with therapy dogs and standardized regulations for safely implementing CAIs across educational contexts. The participants also cited the importance of developing screening protocols to monitor factors that could compromise the safety and welfare of students and the therapy dog-handler team (e.g., dog phobias, therapy dog-handler prior experience and training). The participants also cited the importance of therapy dog-handler training with respect to school-specific challenges (e.g., students who fail to observe protocols for optimal interactions with therapy dogs). Handlers should receive specialized training to work with children and youth who have disabilities or other developmental and mental health challenges that might compromise dog welfare during CAIs. This latter point has been emphasized by CAI researchers and practitioners aiming to safeguard therapy dog welfare within educational contexts (Gee & Fine, 2019;

MacNamara & MacLean, 2017). Additionally, protocols should be established outlining how to handle situations when students fail to observe pre-established rules of engagement that are designed to safe-guard therapy dog welfare (e.g., warnings or restricted/denied access should be applied when a student pulls a dog's tail or ears or handles the dog roughly; Gee & Fine, 2019). Such protocols not only safeguard the welfare of therapy dogs but also ensure the safety of the student clients in CAIs (Meints et al., 2018). In our work at the University of British Columbia (UBC), we ensure that all handlers who participate in our Building Academic Retention Through K9s (B.A.R.K.) program receive training on setting boundaries or *rules of engagement* for how children and youth can safely approach, greet, and interact with their dogs (Binfet & Hartwig, 2020).

ENSURING DOG-HANDLER TEAM WELFARE IN MEDICAL SETTINGS

We also see CAIs being implemented in medical settings ranging from hospitals, dental offices, and medical settings to support human well-being and reduce anxiety among children, adults, and medical

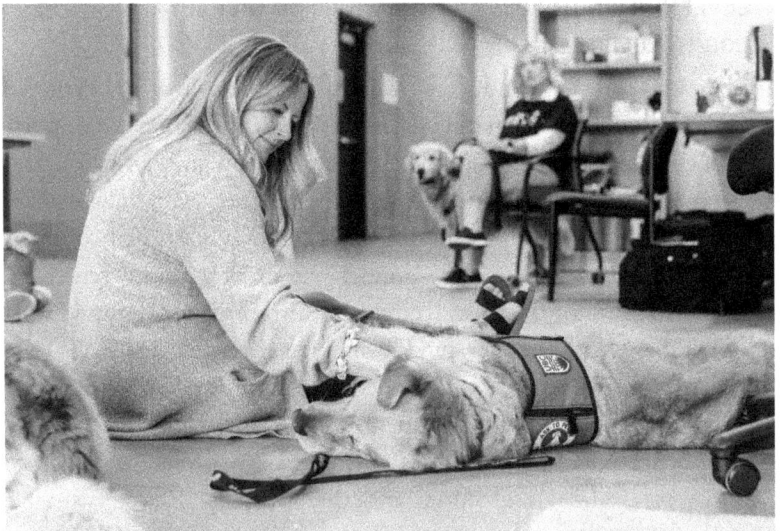

Figure 6.3 Therapy dog Abby, a Golden Retriever, rests comfortably and enjoys receiving physical attention from a client; both the therapy dog and the student are positioned on the floor and appear content
Source: F. L. L. Green Photography; used with permission

residents (e.g., Chubak et al., 2017; Cooley & Barker, 2018; Crossman et al., 2015; Delgado et al., 2018; Harper et al., 2015; Kline et al., 2019; Nammalwar & Rangeeth, 2018; Norton et al., 2018; Schwartz & Patronek, 2002). As is the case with educational settings (see Figure 6.3), medical settings are dynamic, complex, and characterized by unique features that raise important considerations for therapy dog welfare (Barker & Gee, 2021; Townsend & Gee, 2021). Medical settings, particularly hospitals and dentists' offices, include unique stressors for therapy dogs, their handlers, and clients (see Figure 6.4). For instance, these settings often involve bright lights and tiled, slippery flooring; novel and noisy medical equipment; crowding and fast-paced movements, with staff and patients moving around quickly; loud, with frequent, novel, and random sounds (e.g., patient vocalizations of distress, beeping machines, bells, intercom announcements); novel and strong odours (e.g., foods, cleaning agents, bodily fluids); and the expression of intense emotions (e.g., sadness, anxiety and worry) by staff, patients, and visitors (Barker & Gee, 2021; Townsend & Gee, 2021). Patients might also inadvertently cause harm to the therapy dog by handling them too roughly or dropping them due to difficulties with motor skills. Further, environmental changes can unfold rapidly and unexpectedly within medical settings, wherein a relatively calm and quiet evening in an intensive care unit can rapidly turn into a frantic and urgent situation – this quick transition could potentially cause therapy dogs and/or their handlers to become stressed (Table 6.2).

To be sure, medical settings require a great deal of therapy dog-handler team preparation and training (Foss, 2023). Barker and Gee (2021) note that

The handler carries a heavy responsibility in monitoring their dog, their interactions with humans, and any potential risks in the environment. It is important for the CAI program and hospital to provide education and support to handlers in carrying out these responsibilities.

(Barker & Gee, 2021, p. 5)

Further, Foss (2023) argues that the successful implementation of CAIs in healthcare settings rests on several factors including the handlers having in-depth knowledge of the medical environment; training for therapy dog-handler teams that goes beyond what is offered through

Table 6.2 Mitigation Strategies Across Varied Contexts

Environmental Characteristics	Canine Stressors	Handler Contingencies	Mitigation Strategies
• School/classroom • Preschool • Elementary school • Middle school • High school • Gymnasium • University • Library • Community meeting space	• Small children • Unpredictable movements and sounds • Legos, Play-Doh, small toys that dogs could eat; things with wheels • Balls of different sizes (some bigger than dog) • Food and snacks that children want to feed them • Unregistered dogs may have different levels of training and tolerance for animal-assisted education • Slippery flooring • Demands for continual movement • Other classroom pets (hamster, gerbil)	• Pressure to meet educational goal • Crowd control • Navigating unfamiliar environment • Ever-changing environment (school hallways, classroom decorations) • Divided attentional demands if handler is also the teacher	Proactive education about how to interact with dog Additional advocates to serve as "buffer" Pre-event visit to familiarize dog with setting Plan in advance to clear the floor of debris Train children how to interact with dogs Provide space for those who do not want to interact with dog Involve a classroom aide if teacher is serving as handler

Source: Townsend & Gee, 2021; used with permission from *Veterinary Sciences*

therapy dog registering organizations to include the unique considerations of healthcare settings and diverse patient profiles; training for all individuals involved including staff, patients, visitors, and volunteers; and awareness and understanding of animal enjoyment and stress indicators in CAIs within medical contexts. Here, too, it's important to develop screening protocols to monitor factors that could compromise the safety and welfare of staff, patients, and the therapy dog-handler team, and to develop standardized regulations for safely implementing CAIs across medical contexts.

WELFARE CONSIDERATIONS IN CORRECTIONAL FACILITIES

Another context in which we see CAIs being implemented is within prisons and correctional facilities to develop empathy skills and to support social skills and well-being among adults and incarcerated youth (e.g., Allison & Ramaswamy, 2016; Chalmers et al., 2023; Conniff et al., 2005; Dell et al., 2019a, 2019b; Fournier et al., 2007; Gibson et al., 2023; Harbolt & Ward, 2001; Kosteniuk et al., 2023; Seivert et al., 2018; Smith et al., 2023; Strimple, 2003). These canine-assistance dogs in the justice system are sometimes referred to as *cell dogs* (Duindam et al., 2021). *Cell dogs* are often paired with adults and incarcerated youth to develop new skills such as dog training, to develop human-animal bonds, or to *create canine and relational connections*. As an example, Colleen Dell from the University of Saskatchewan, along with her colleagues, is forging new empirical terrain and offering insights into how therapy dogs can benefit incarcerated individuals (see *About the PAWSitive connections lab*, n.d; Dell et al., 2019a, 2019b; Gibson et al., 2023) (Figure 6.4).

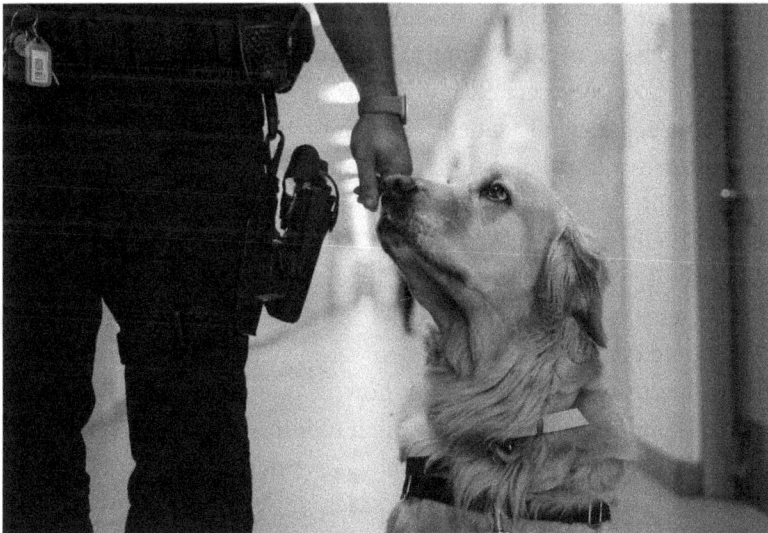

Figure 6.4 Abby, a therapy dog, looks up at a police officer as they walk side by side down a hallway
Source: Freya L. L. Green Photography; used with permission

Prisons and correctional facilities are dynamic and characterized by unique features that raise important considerations for therapy dog welfare (Eaton-Stull, 2022). Therapy dog-handler teams can face several types of stressors when they participate in CAIs within prisons and correctional facilities. As is the case in medical contexts, these settings often involve bright lights and tiled, slippery flooring; loud and random sounds (e.g., client vocalizations of distress, intercom announcements); novel and strong odours (e.g., foods, cleaning agents, bodily fluids, firearms); and the expression of intense emotions (e.g., anxiety, concern, anger, sadness) by staff, clients, and visitors. Also, environmental changes can unfold rapidly and unexpectedly in these settings. A relatively calm and quiet evening in a correctional facility can rapidly turn into a chaotic situation when an incarcerated youth experiences a mental health crisis characterized by shouting and aggressive behaviours. These sudden transitions and the environmental features of prisons and correctional facilities could potentially cause therapy dogs and/or their handlers to become stressed. Visiting a prison or correctional facility can be a stressful experience. Handlers might become anxious, and as we discussed in Chapter 5, a handler's anxious feelings could travel down the leash and cause their dog to become stressed through a process of emotional contagion.

Clients' profiles and their past experiences with dogs (and animals) should also be considered when safeguarding therapy dog welfare. For instance, some incarcerated individuals might exhibit impulsive and aggressive behavioural tendencies, express intense emotions, and/or have histories of self-harm or harming dogs (animals). An incarcerated youth might, unexpectedly, harm a therapy dog by pushing it aside or pulling its tail. It is the responsibility of handlers and prison or correctional facility personnel to prepare for such contingencies in advance of a CAI session (Eaton-Stull, 2022). The design and implementation of CAIs should consider clients' past animal-related experiences and offer some education in advance about how to interact with therapy dogs optimally and respectfully. Behavioural training might be required for prison inmates and youth involved in the criminal justice system who show aggressive behavioural tendencies or who have past negative experiences with animals, and their interactions with therapy dogs may require continual monitoring. Recall the scenario at the outset of this chapter: Arya should be required to collect information about the young people in his care and their past experiences with dogs (animals) and receive training prior to introducing them to a therapy dog. In turn, Arya should consult with the therapy dog handler in advance to develop a plan to educate and instruct the youth on how best to interact with the therapy dog to optimize the dog's agency and enjoyment throughout the session. As discussed in Chapters 3 and 5, the youth should also learn about therapy dog consent in advance of the first visit.

DOG-HANDLER TEAM WELFARE IN VIRTUAL CONTEXTS

Researchers are currently exploring the promise of virtual interactions with dog-handler teams to support human health and well-being (for a review, see Tardif-Williams & Binfet, 2023). Virtual CAIs create new and exciting opportunities for geographically and sociodemographically diverse clients to interact with therapy dog-handler teams. A distinct advantage of virtual CAIs for human clients is that they can engage people who are living in geographically remote locations where opportunities to interact with therapy dog-handler teams are limited. This might include incarcerated youth in a correctional facility; people who have allergies, fears, or histories of aggression towards animals that make interacting with therapy dogs impossible or challenging; and people who are reluctant to receive mental health services. In turn, virtual CAIs occur in relatively unobtrusive spaces wherein therapy dog-handler teams can be observed, and therapy dog agency and welfare can be more easily privileged and optimized. In this way, professionals and researchers working with diverse clients could leverage virtual CAIs to support human health and well-being and promote a responsible and compassionate ethic towards therapy dogs (and animals). Virtual CAIs might be a particularly attractive first option for Arya who is considering how to create connections between therapy dogs and incarcerated youth in a correctional facility, as some of the youth might find it challenging to regulate intense emotions (e.g., anger outbursts) or have histories of animal cruelty. Also, virtual interactions buffer therapy dog stress by reducing overwork since there is no direct contact or hands-on interactions between the dog and the client. Virtual contexts might be ideal for optimizing welfare for therapy dogs who do not enjoy participating in CAIs (Ein et al., 2022). Note, however, that while this might be the case, our research indicates that engaging in virtual CAIs can also be taxing and draining on therapy dogs and their handlers in unique ways. Drawing on our own and other's published research on developing and implementing virtual CAIs to support students' well-being and learning (Binfet et al., 2022a; Dell et al., 2021; Steel, 2023; Tardif-Williams et al., 2023), we consider some of the challenges that can compromise therapy dog welfare in a virtual context and offer recommendations for best practices in optimizing therapy dog-handler team welfare and enjoyment in virtual settings (Figure 6.5).

Creating and implementing virtual CAIs involves unique elements that raise considerations for therapy dog welfare (Tardif-Williams & Binfet, 2023). Therapy dog-handler teams can face several types of stressors when they participate in virtual CAIs including heat from additional lighting; bright lights and tiled, slippery flooring; having to hold steady in one position for lengthy periods to remain in the viewing frame; new and unfamiliar environments including having to sit or stand on an elevated platform to facilitate videography sessions; new and unfamiliar faces moving about the space; and novel and noisy video equipment. Within virtual contexts, the handler must

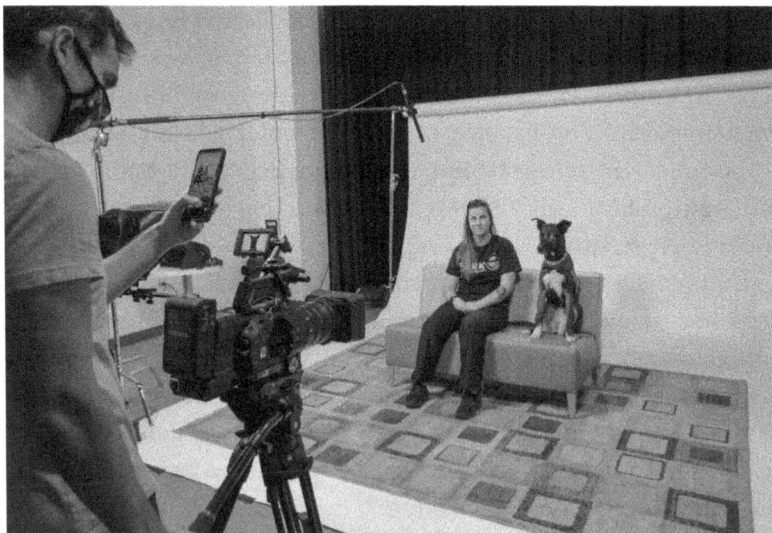

Figure 6.5 Videographer Taylor, handler Ty, and her therapy dog Luna from UBC's B.A.R.K. program preparing for a filming session in a studio
Source: Freya L. L. Green Photography; used with permission

simultaneously monitor their dog's welfare and oversee various challenges including keeping their dog within the viewing frame when filming, following a script, and responding to clients and their questions when virtual interactions unfold in real time. Attending to these challenges might compromise the handler's ability to monitor and advocate for their dog's welfare, as their focus is divided. Further, virtual contexts may be less rewarding and satisfying for therapy dog-handler teams who enjoy interacting and forming bonds with other people and therapy dogs (Rousseau et al., 2020).

We recommend having handler training or practice sessions wherein handlers and their dogs can become familiar with the technology and the filming space and making program personnel available to assist with technology and filming. This will allow the therapy dog-handler team to become comfortable with the procedures and processes and will support each handler's ability to simultaneously monitor their dog's welfare and enjoyment during virtual sessions. We also recommend having experienced welfare monitors available

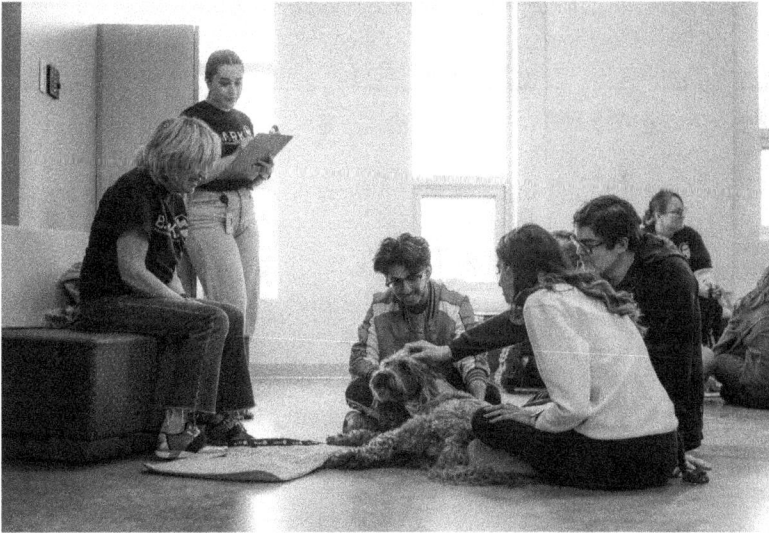

Figure 6.6 A group of university students sitting on the ground engaging with therapy dog Cali and her handler. Madisyn, an experienced monitor, stands nearby to assess the dog's welfare and enjoyment; the handler has instructed the students to sit in a way that allows for a clear exit path
Source: F. L. L. Green Photography; used with permission

Table 6.3 Welfare Checklist

1	Have the animal and handler undergone screening to determine suitability for the work in question? (i.e., has the animal's potential to participate in virtual human-animal connections been assessed?)
2	If supplemental lighting is used to support the quality of filming, is the temperature being monitored to prevent animals overheating?
3	Is water available before, during, and after filming?
4	Has the human participant been provided instruction/education regarding how to optimally interact?
5	Have efforts been made to obtain consent from the animal?
6	Does the interaction encourage the animal to demonstrate natural behaviors?
7	Is the animal determining participation and able to voluntarily cease to participate?
8	Is the duration of the intervention and the number of interventions per day in accordance with recommended best practices?
9	Have time-out breaks be scheduled as part of each working session?
10	Have barriers or deterrents to reporting adverse effects been acknowledged/recognized? (i.e., reflecting poorly on the agency)
11	Is there a designated human responsible for the welfare advocacy of the animal? If not, how will the handler monitor welfare whilst concurrently overseeing the virtual human animal interaction session?

Source: Tardif-Williams & Binfet, 2023; used with permission from Routledge

to assist each handler in monitoring their dog's welfare during virtual sessions; this will reduce the burden placed on handlers, help to optimize therapy dog welfare, and enhance the therapy dog-handler team's ability to support clients. Here, too, it's important to develop screening protocols to monitor factors that could compromise the safety and welfare of the therapy dog-handler team and to develop standardized regulations for safely creating and actualizing CAIs in virtual contexts (Figure 6.6). See Table 6.3 for a list of considerations for therapy dogs (animals) participating in virtual contexts.

WELFARE CONSIDERATIONS WITH SPECIALIZED POPULATIONS IN SPECIALIZED CONTEXTS

As previously noted, CAIs have surged in popularity, and we now see therapy dog-handler teams placed in a variety of public and specialized settings to support the health and well-being of diverse clients. In addition to educational, medical, correctional, and virtual contexts, we see therapy dog-handler teams placed in airports, crisis response settings (e.g., environmental disasters, school or workplace tragedies, and to support first responders), funeral homes, shelters for people experiencing homelessness, long-term care facilities, police detachments and military bases, and public libraries (for a review, see Binfet & Hartwig, 2020). Increasingly, we also see therapy dog-handler teams supporting human health and well-being as part of workplace innovations (Foreman et al., 2017; Hall et al., 2017; Hall & Mills, 2019; Junça-Silva, 2022; Wagner et al., 2021) and recreational programs such as *puppy or dog yoga* (e.g., *How puppy yoga is helping people with anxiety*, 2022; *Downward dog is easy in this pup-filled yoga class*, 2023).

It merits noting that within these public and specialized settings CAIs can unfold in especially dynamic and unpredictable ways, thus heightening concerns for therapy dog-handler welfare. For instance, crisis response settings (e.g., environmental disasters, school or workplace tragedies) can involve intense emotions for therapy dog-handler teams. These settings are often characterized by large numbers of people and fast-paced and chaotic movements and therapy dog-handler teams might be invited to participate in lengthier sessions across several days. Further, therapy dog-handler teams can also face intense emotions when they support first responders following their involvement in a crisis response situation; first responders might be experiencing heightened anxiety and other post-traumatic stress-related symptoms. Therapy dog-handler teams might also face intense emotions when they support grieving people in funeral home settings. These features of crisis response and funeral settings make therapy dog-handler teams especially vulnerable to overwork and stress, and additional care needs to be taken to safeguard their welfare. Townsend and Gee (2021) recommend providing frequent breaks and adjusting the intensity, duration, and frequency of therapy dog-handler sessions in crisis response settings to minimize dogs' experience of stress. It is also important to note that not all therapy dog-handler teams are suitable for participation in this type of high-intensity environment. Therapy dog-handler teams should undergo specialized training and screening for suitability (i.e., overall flexibility and resiliency) to assist in environments characterized by unpredictability and emotional intensity (Eaton-Stull & Flynn, 2015). As discussed in previous chapters, emotional contagion is an important issue to consider in emotionally intense settings as clients' and/or handlers' emotions could travel down the leash and cause a therapy dog to become stressed. Handlers intimately know their dog's typical behaviours and preferences, playing a critical role in continuously monitoring and advocating for their dog's welfare in these highly complex and unpredictable environments. To optimize their dog's welfare, handlers can provide more frequent breaks, reduce the number of sessions, or discontinue participation.

Therapy dog handlers also face unique welfare considerations when they support human health and well-being within recreational and workplace settings. For instance, these settings often involve large numbers of diverse people and, depending on the type of workplace setting or recreation, can include novel and noisy equipment, fast-paced movements, and loud and unpredictable sounds. For instance, therapy dog-handler teams supporting multiple clients at a busy airport will experience a much noisier and more energetic environment, as compared to therapy dog-handler teams supporting a smaller group of staff and senior clients at a long-term care facility. Some workplace and recreational settings also include multiple therapy dog-handler teams or non-therapy dogs, and this can raise safety and welfare considerations for therapy dog-handler teams. Recently, a spotlight has been focused on the welfare concerns associated with dog yoga which has become an increasingly popular form of physical recreation. Welfare concerns include taking puppies away from their mothers at a young age; overcrowding and potential injury; inadequate rest and water breaks; and lack of monitors to oversee dog's welfare and enjoyment (e.g., RSPCA urges animal-lovers to say no to puppy yoga classes, 2023; Dunne, 2023).

As is the case with more structured CAIs, handlers should take precautions in advance to ensure that these settings will be suitable for their dog's energy levels and preferences for personal space, proximity to other dogs, type and number of clients, and length, duration, and frequency of sessions. Also, efforts should be made to prepare clients in the workplace or recreational setting by offering education on how to optimally interact with the dog, and rules of engagement and boundaries should be established. Both handlers and staff share the responsibility of preparing clients for interactions with therapy dogs and for continuously monitoring therapy dog welfare during canine-assisted sessions. As is the case with more structured CAIs, therapy dogs' agency, welfare, and enjoyment must be prioritized and optimized within CAIs involving specialized settings and clients.

CAI Research as a Specialized Context

It merits noting that participation in CAI research constitutes a specialized context requiring therapy dog-handler teams to collaborate with several team members including researchers and research assistants, volunteer students, teachers, medical staff, and diverse study participants. Therapy dog-handler teams might also be required to assist in diverse environments ranging from strictly controlled laboratories to more naturalistic settings such as university campuses, public libraries, and hospitals. As part of research procedures, therapy dogs might be required to momentarily inhibit some of their preferences (e.g., playful behaviours), remain in a specified position for longer than is desired, perform repetitive tasks, and engage with multiple participants and sometimes for lengthy sessions. These features of research contexts make therapy dog-handler teams especially vulnerable to overwork and stress, and additional care needs to be taken to safeguard their welfare. Certainly, our research in designing and offering CAIs to varied client populations indicates that not all therapy dog-handler teams are ideally suitable for participation in research contexts. We recommend that therapy dog-handler teams undergo specialized training and screening for suitability to assist in research contexts that are often characterized by pre-specified and sequenced procedures.

In Chapter 3, we noted that researchers are required to receive institutional clearance from research ethics boards when they engage in research with animal and human participants. We argued that this is a necessary but insufficient condition for safeguarding therapy dog-handler team welfare in research contexts. Additionally, it is the responsibility of handlers, researchers, and program personnel to ensure that therapy dog welfare is actualized within dynamic and specialized research contexts throughout all phases of the research process. In Chapter 3, we noted that this can be particularly problematic for researchers and therapy dog handlers who are committed to the successful execution of a research study. Moving forward, we reiterate our call for researchers to prioritize dog-handler team welfare and enjoyment within CAI research. Therapy dog-handler team welfare and enjoyment within CAI research are integral to increasing methodological rigour and, ultimately, the validity of research results.

Dog-Handler Teams Supporting Unique and Vulnerable Populations

As the fields of animal-assisted intervention (AAI) and CAI expand and the demand to interact with therapy dogs grows, we see dog-handler teams volunteer in settings and in support of clients that extends beyond the typical settings of retirement homes or university campuses. Dog-handler teams may be asked to work in specialized settings (e.g., police detachment) where advanced training is required around how best to support clients while safeguarding their dogs' welfare. It is the responsibility of the larger therapy dog organization to provide this specialized training and ensure that teams are well suited and equipped to work in such a capacity. Recognizing that not all dogs are suited to working in all environments and with all clients, we might see dog-handler teams with unique or nuanced expertise (e.g., working with hospitalized children). That is, the combination of the handler's skills and the dog's temperament and interest in working with specific populations might see the team better suited to volunteer in one setting over other settings. Take, for example, dog-handler teams working in prison settings to support the well-being of incarcerated individuals. Not all handlers and not all dogs would be well suited to volunteering within this specialized context.

We recognize that, to some extent, all contexts in which CAIs unfold are specialized. For dog-handler teams to volunteer in specialized settings, it is recommended they have ample prior experience volunteering in traditional settings in support of typical clients – in this regard, the team may build and hone their skills and build capacity for more nuanced work. Ideally, we recommend that therapy dog-handler teams first develop and practice their skills in a relatively calming context with a small number of clients, preferably with one or two clients at a time. As therapy dog-handler teams gain experience and confidence, they could be invited to participate in a more specialized contexts and with specialized clients. For instance, a novice therapy dog-handler team might not be ready to dive into a crisis response setting or to interact with children who have attention-deficit hyperactivity disorder. However, as discussed in Chapter 5, with experience and ongoing training relevant to these latter settings and clients therapy dog-handler teams gain confidence, handlers are better able to advocate for their dog's welfare and the dog-handler team is better able to support human clients.

CONCLUSION

As the field of CAIs broadens and extends its reach, we see therapy dog-handler teams being placed in a variety of new contexts in support of new and diverse clients. This chapter challenged readers to reconsider therapy dog-handler team welfare within challenging, dynamic, and applied contexts replete with several unknown and ever-changing variables. We reviewed the varied contexts and the diverse clients supported, to date, by CAIs, and we discussed welfare considerations across these contexts (i.e., from educational, medical, and correctional facilities to virtual settings). In Chapter 7, we discuss specific practices and measures that can be established in advance of CAIs to help ensure the safety and welfare of both therapy dogs and their handlers. Considerations here include insurance liability coverage, an ecological assessment of the setting dog-handler teams work in, and the importance of documenting and reporting incidents of compromised welfare.

REFERENCES

About the PAWSitive connections lab. (n.d.). Pawsitiveconnectionslab.Com. Retrieved June 14, 2024, from https://pawsitiveconnectionslab.com/

Allison, M., & Ramaswamy, M. (2016). Adapting animal-assisted therapy trials to prison-based animal programs. *Public Health Nursing, 33*(5), 472–480. https://doi.org/10.1111/phn.12276

Bailey, K. (2023). A scoping review of campus-based animal-assisted interactions programs for college student mental health. *People and Animals: The International Journal of Research and Practice, 6*(1) 1–27. https://doi.org/10.62845/iqjlqog

Baird, R., Berger, E., & Grové, C. (2023). Therapy dogs and school wellbeing: A qualitative study. *Journal of Veterinary Behavior, 68*, 15–23. https://doi.org/10.1016/j.jveb.2023.08.005

Baird, R., Grové, C., & Berger, E. (2022). The impact of therapy dogs on the social and emotional wellbeing of students: A systematic review. *Educational and Developmental Psychologist, 39*(2), 180–208. https://doi.org/10.1080/20590776.2022.2049444

Barker, S. B., Barker, R. T., McCain, N. L., & Schubert, C. M. (2016). A randomized cross-over exploratory study of the effect of visiting therapy dogs on college student stress before final exams. *Anthrozoös, 29*(1), 35–46. https://doi.org/10.1080/08927936.2015.1069988

Barker, S. B., & Gee, N. R. (2021). Canine-assisted interventions in hospitals: Best practices for maximizing human and canine safety. *Frontiers in Veterinary Science, 8*, 1–12. https://doi.org/10.3389/fvets.2021.615730

Binfet, J. T. (2017). The effects of group-administered canine therapy on university students' wellbeing: A randomized controlled trial. *Anthrozoös, 30*(3), 397–414. https://doi.org/10.1080/08927936.2017.1335097

Binfet, J. T., Green, F. L., & Draper, Z. A. (2022a). The importance of client–canine contact in canine-assisted interventions: A randomized controlled trial. *Anthrozoös, 35*(1), 1–22. https://doi.org/10.1080/08927936.2021.1944558

Binfet, J. T., & Hartwig, E. K. (2020). *Canine-assisted interventions: A comprehensive guide to credentialing therapy dog teams.* Routledge.

Binfet, J. T., Passmore, H.-A., Cebry, A., Struik, K., & McKay, C. (2018). Reducing university students' stress through a drop-in canine-therapy program. *Journal of Mental Health, 27*(3), 197–204. https://doi.org/10.1080/09638237.2017.1417551

Bremhorst, A., & Mills, D. (2021). Working with companion animals, and especially dogs, in therapeutic and other AAI settings. In J. M. Peralta & A. Fine (Eds.), *The welfare of animals in animal-assisted interventions: Foundations and best practice methods* (pp. 191–217). Springer.

Chalmers, D., Dell, C., Dixon, J., & Rath, G. (2023). PAWSitive support: A canine assisted learning program to support prisoners in healing from substance use. In R. Ciernick, W. Rowe, & G. Novotna (Eds.), *Responding to the oppression of addiction* (4th ed., p. 451). Canadian Scholars.

Chubak, J., Hawkes, R., Dudzik, C., Foose-Foster, J. M., Eaton, L., Johnson, R. H., & Macpherson, C. F. (2017). Pilot study of therapy dog visits for inpatient youth with cancer. *Journal of Pediatric Oncology Nursing, 34*(5), 331–341. https://doi.org/10.1177/1043454217712983

Conniff, K. M., Scarlett, J. M., Goodman, S., & Appel, L. D. (2005). Effects of a pet visitation program on the behavior and emotional state of adjudicated female adolescents. *Anthrozoös, 18*(4), 379–395. https://doi.org/10.2752/089279305785593974

Cooley, L. F., & Barker, S. B. (2018). Canine-assisted therapy as an adjunct tool in the care of the surgical patient: A literature review and opportunity for research. *Alternative Therapies in Health and Medicine, 24*(3), 48–51.

Crossman, M. K., Kazdin, A. E., & Knudson, K. (2015). Brief unstructured interaction with a dog reduces distress. *Anthrozoös, 28*(4), 649–659. https://doi.org/10.1080/08927936.2015.1070008

Delgado, C., Toukonen, M., & Wheeler, C. (2018). Effect of canine play interventions as a stress reduction strategy in college students. *Nurse Educator, 43*(3), 149–153. https://doi.org/10.1097/nne.0000000000000451

Dell, C, Chalmers, D., Cole, D., & Dixon, J. (2019a). Prisoners accessing relational connections with dogs: A just outcome of the St. John Ambulance therapy dog program at Stony Mountain Institution. In S. Kohm, K. Walby, K. Gorkoff, & K. Maier (Eds.), *The annual review of interdisciplinary justice research* (Vol. 8, pp. 14–64). The University of Winnipeg Centre for Interdisciplinary Justice Studies (CIJS).

Dell, C., Chalmers, D., Stobbe, M., Rohr, B., & Husband, A. (2019b). Animal-assisted therapy in a Canadian psychiatric prison. *International Journal of Prisoner Health, 15*(3), 209–231. https://doi.org/10.1108/ijph-04-2018-0020

Dell, C., Williamson, L., McKenzie, H., Carey, B., Cruz, M., Gibson, M., & Pavelich, A. (2021). A commentary about lessons learned: Transitioning a therapy dog program online during the COVID-19 pandemic. *Animals*, 11(3), 914. https://doi.org/10.3390/ani11030914

Downward dog is easy in this pup-filled yoga class. (2023, January 28). BBC News. https://www.bbc.com/news/av/world-us-canada-64417730

Dunne, J. (2023, October 21). *Puppy yoga is the latest wellness trend – is it a good thing?*. Vet Help Direct. https://vethelpdirect.com/vetblog/2023/10/21/puppy-yoga-is-the-latest-wellness-trend-is-it-a-good-thing/

Duindam, H. M., Creemers, H. E., Hoeve, M., & Asscher, J. J. (2021). Breaking the chains? The effects of training a shelter dog in prison on criminal behavior and recidivism. *Applied Developmental Science*, 26(4), 813–826. https://doi.org/10.1080/10888691.2021.2007768

Eaton-Stull, Y. (2022). Animal-assisted social work in prisons. In L. Rapp-McCall, K. Corcoran, & A. R. Roberts (Eds.), *Social workers' desk reference* (4th ed., pp. 1307–1313). Oxford University Press.

Eaton-Stull, Y., & Flynn, B. (2015). Animal-assisted crisis response. In K. R. Yeager & A. R. Roberts (Eds.), *Crisis intervention handbook: Assessment, treatment, and research* (4th ed., pp. 599–606). Oxford University Press.

Ein, N., Gervasio, J., Reed, M. J., & Vickers, K. (2022). Effects on wellbeing of exposure to dog videos before a stressor. *Anthrozoös*, 36(3), 349–367. https://doi.org/10.1080/08927936.2022.2149925

Fine, A. H. (2019). *Handbook on animal-assisted therapy: Foundations and guidelines for animal-assisted interventions*. Academic Press.

Foreman, A., Glenn, M., Meade, B., & Wirth, O. (2017). Dogs in the workplace: A review of the benefits and potential challenges. *International Journal of Environmental Research and Public Health*, 14(5), 498. https://doi.org/10.3390/ijerph14050498

Foss, C. (2023). Welfare and safety considerations in AAI hospital programs. *Animal-Assisted Interventions*, 130–131. https://doi.org/10.1079/9781800622616.0029

Fournier, A. K., Geller, E. S., & Fortney, E. V. (2007). Human-animal interaction in a prison setting: Impact on criminal behavior, treatment progress, and social skills. *Behavior and Social Issues*, 16(1), 89–105. https://doi.org/10.5210/bsi.v16i1.385

Gee, N. R., & Fine, A. (2019). Animals in educational settings: Research and application. In A. Fine (Ed.), *Animal assisted therapy: Theoretical foundations and guidelines for practice* (5th ed.). Academic Press.

Gee, N. R., Griffin, J. A., & McCardle, P. (2017). Human–animal interaction research in school settings: Current knowledge and future directions. *AERA Open*, 3(3), 1–9. https://doi.org/10.1177/2332858417724346

Gibson, M., Dell, C. A., Chalmers, D., Rath, G., & Mela, M. (2023). Unleashing compassionate care: Canine-assisted intervention as a promising harm reduction approach to prisonization in Canada and its relevance to forensic psychiatry. *Frontiers in Psychiatry*, 14, 1–7. https://doi.org/10.3389/fpsyt.2023.1219096

Glenk, L. (2017). Current perspectives on therapy dog welfare in animal-assisted interventions. *Animals*, 7(12), 7. https://doi.org/10.3390/ani7020007

Grové, C., Henderson, L., Lee, F., & Wardlaw, P. (2021). Therapy dogs in educational settings: Guidelines and recommendations for implementation. *Frontiers in Veterinary Science*, 8, 1–14. https://doi.org/10.3389/fvets.2021.655104

Hall, S. S., & Mills, D. S. (2019). Taking dogs into the office: A novel strategy for promoting work engagement, commitment and quality of life. *Frontiers in Veterinary Science*, 6, 1–17. https://doi.org/10.3389/fvets.2019.00138

Hall, S., Wright, H., McCune, S., Zulch, H., & Mills, D. (2017). Perceptions of dogs in the workplace: The pros and the cons. *Anthrozoös*, 30(2), 291–305. https://doi.org/10.1080/08927936.2017.1311053

Harbolt, T., & Ward, T. (2001). Teaming incarcerated youth with shelter dogs for a second chance. *Society & Animals*, 9(2), 177–182. https://doi.org/10.1163/156853001753639279

Harper, C. M., Dong, Y., Thornhill, T. S., Wright, J., Ready, J., Brick, G. W., & Dyer, G. (2015). Can therapy dogs improve pain and satisfaction after total joint arthroplasty? A randomized controlled trial. *Clinical Orthopaedics and Related Research*, 473(1), 372–379. https://doi.org/10.1007/s11999-014-3931-0

How puppy yoga is helping people with anxiety. (2022, November 14). BBC News. https://www.bbc.com/news/av/uk-england-manchester-63625957

Junça-Silva, A. (2022). Friends with benefits: The positive consequences of pet-friendly practices for workers' well-being. *International Journal of Environmental Research and Public Health*, 19(3), 1069. https://doi.org/10.3390/ijerph19031069

King, C., Watters, J., & Mungre, S. (2011). Effect of a time-out session with working animal-assisted therapy dogs. *Journal of Veterinary Behavior*, 6(4), 232–238. https://doi.org/10.1016/j.jveb.2011.01.007

Kirnan, J., Siminerio, S., & Wong, Z. (2016). The impact of a therapy dog program on children's reading skills and attitudes toward reading. *Early Childhood Education Journal*, 44(6), 637–651. https://doi.org/10.1007/s10643-015-0747-9

Kivlen, C., Winston, K., Mills, D., DiZazzo-Miller, R., Davenport, R., & Binfet, J.-T. (2022). Canine-assisted intervention effects on the well-being of health science graduate students: A randomized controlled trial. *The American Journal of Occupational Therapy*, 76(6), https://doi.org/10.5014/ajot.2022.049508

Kline, J. A., Fisher, M. A., Pettit, K. L., Linville, C. T., & Beck, A. M. (2019). Controlled clinical trial of canine therapy versus usual care to reduce patient anxiety in the emergency department. *PLOS ONE*, 14(1), 1–13. https://doi.org/10.1371/journal.pone.0209232

Kosteniuk, B., Dell, C. A., Cruz, M., & Chalmers, D. (2023). An experiential approach to canine-assisted learning in corrections for prisoners who use substances. *Journal of Forensic Nursing*, 19(3), 197–203. https://doi.org/10.1097/jfn.0000000000000435

MacNamara, M., & MacLean, E. (2017). Selecting animals for education environments. In Nancy R. Gee, Aubrey H. Fine, Peggy McCardle (Eds.), *How animals help students learn: Research and practice for educators and mental-health professionals* (pp. 182–196). Taylor and Francis.

Marinelli, L., Normando, S., Siliprandi, C., Salvadoretti, M., & Mongillo, P. (2009). Dog assisted interventions in a specialized centre and potential concerns for animal welfare. *Veterinary Research Communication*, 33, 93–95.

Meints, K., Brelsford, V., & De Keuster, T. (2018). Teaching children and parents to understand dog signaling. *Frontiers in Veterinary Science*, 5, 1–14. https://doi.org/10.3389/fvets.2018.00257

Nammalwar, R., & Rangeeth, P. (2018). A bite out of anxiety: Evaluation of animal-assisted activity on anxiety in children attending a pediatric dental outpatient unit. *Journal of Indian Society of Pedodontics and Preventive Dentistry*, 36(2), 181. https://doi.org/10.4103/jisppd.jisppd_54_18

Norton, M. J., Funaro, M. C., & Rojiani, R. (2018). Improving healthcare professionals' well-being through the use of therapy dogs. *Journal of Hospital Librarianship*, 18(3), 203–209. https://doi.org/10.1080/15323269.2018.1471898

Pendry, P., Carr, A. M., Roeter, S. M., & Vandagriff, J. L. (2018). Experimental trial demonstrates effects of animal-assisted stress prevention program on college students' positive and negative emotion. *Human-Animal Interaction Bulletin*, 6(1), 81–97. https://doi.org/10.1079/hai.2018.0004

Pendry, P., & Vandagriff, J. L. (2019). Animal visitation program (AVP) reduces cortisol levels of university students: A randomized controlled trial. *AERA Open*, 5(2), 1–12. https://doi.org/10.1177/2332858419852592

Reilly, K. M., Adesope, O. O., & Erdman, P. (2020). The effects of dogs on learning: A meta-analysis. *Anthrozoös*, 33(3), 339–360. https://doi.org/10.1080/08927936.2020.1746523

Renck Jalongo, M., & Petro, J. (2018). Promoting children's well-being: Therapy dogs. *Children, Dogs and Education*, 179–209. https://doi.org/10.1007/978-3-319-77845-7_9

Rousseau, C. X., Binfet, J.-T., Green, F. I. L., Tardif-Williams, C. Y., Draper, Z. A., & Maynard, A. (2020). Up the leash: Exploring canine handlers' perceptions of volunteering in canine-assisted interventions. *Pet Behaviour Science*, 10(10), 15–35. https://doi.org/10.21071/pbs.vi10.12598

Rousseau, C. X., & Tardif-Williams, C. Y. (2019). Turning the page for Spot: The potential of therapy dogs to support reading motivation among young children. *Anthrozoös*, 32(5), 665–677. https://doi.org/10.1080/08927936.2019.1645511

RSPCA urges animal-lovers to say no to puppy yoga classes. RSPCA. (2023). https://www.rspca.org.uk/-/news-rspca-urges-animal-lovers-to-say-no-to-puppy-yoga-classes

Sandt, D. D. (2020). Effective implementation of animal assisted education interventions in the inclusive early childhood education classroom. *Early Childhood Education Journal*, 48(1), 103–115. https://doi.org/10.1007/s10643-019-01000-z

Schwartz, A., & Patronek, G. (2002). Methodological issues in studying the anxiety-reducing effects of animals: Reflections from a pediatric dental study. *Anthrozoös*, 15(4), 290–299. https://doi.org/10.2752/089279302786992432

Seivert, N. P., Cano, A., Casey, R. J., May, D. K., & Johnson, A. (2018). Animal assisted therapy for incarcerated youth: A randomized controlled trial. *Applied Developmental Science*, 22(2), 139–153. https://doi.org/10.1080/10888691.2016.1234935

Smith, S., Dell, C. A., Claypool, T., Chalmers, D., & Khalid, A. (2023). Case report: A community case study of the human-animal bond in animal-assisted therapy: The experiences of psychiatric prisoners with therapy dogs. *Frontiers in Psychiatry*, 14, 1–10. https://doi.org/10.3389/fpsyt.2023.1219305

Steel, J. (2023). Reading to dogs in schools: A controlled feasibility study of an online reading to dogs intervention. *International Journal of Educational Research*, 117, 102117. https://doi.org/10.1016/j.ijer.2022.102117

Strimple, E. O. (2003). A history of prison inmate-animal interaction programs. *American Behavioral Scientist*, 47(1), 70–78. https://doi.org/10.1177/0002764203255212

Tardif-Williams, C. Y., & Binfet, J.-T. (2023). Virtual human-animal interactions. *Routledge*. https://doi.org/10.4324/9781003327868

Townsend, L., & Gee, N. R. (2021). Recognizing and mitigating canine stress during animal assisted interventions. *Veterinary Sciences*, 8(11), 254. https://doi.org/10.3390/vetsci8110254

Wagner, E., & Pina e Cunha, M. (2021). Dogs at the workplace: A multiple case study. *Animals*, 11(1), 89. https://doi.org/10.3390/ani11010089

Winkle, M., Johnson, A., & Mills, D. (2020). Dog welfare, well-being and behavior: Considerations for selection, evaluation and suitability for animal-assisted therapy. *Animals*, 10(11), 2188. https://doi.org/10.3390/ani10112188

Wood, E., Ohlsen, S., Thompson, J., Hulin, J., & Knowles, L. (2018). The feasibility of brief dog-assisted therapy on university students stress levels: The paws study. *Journal of Mental Health*, 27(3), 263–268. https://doi.org/10.1080/09638237.2017.1385737

Seven

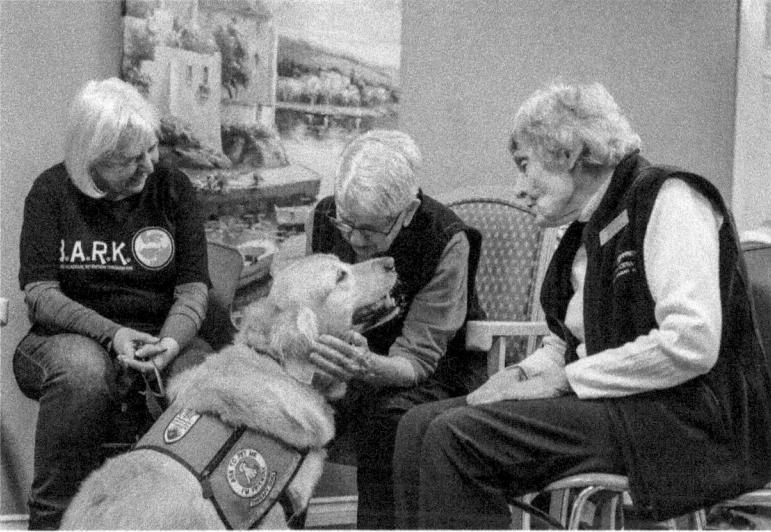

Figure 7.1 Volunteer handler Maureen facilitates a visit between her therapy dog Dash and seniors in a residential care facility

Source: Freya L. L. Green Photography; used with permission

DOI: 10.4324/9781032639284-7

SCENARIO

I Was Only Gone for a Minute

Looking around the retirement facility, all was quiet. There were but a few regular residents who'd come to this week's session. Needing to use the restroom, Cindy asked Marla, a long-time resident and frequent visitor to the Dogs in Residence program at Shady Shores Retirement Facility, to watch her dog Jack as she ran to the restroom. Upon her return, Marla and Jack were nowhere in sight; Cindy's heart was skipping a beat. Clear across the facility and in the cafeteria, Cindy saw Marla leading Jack between tables of residents gathered for a mid-morning coffee and snack, and residents offering Jack tidbits from their plates. Before she could intervene, the facility manager was seen escorting Marla by the elbow out of the cafeteria, Jack in tow (Figure 7.1). "I'd just run to the restroom," explained Cindy to which the manager replied: "Isn't there a policy forbidding residents from walking therapy dogs? Remember Mrs. Campbell is deathly afraid of dogs – that's why we have the dog program stationed over by the recreation room. It's best to get a staff member to cover for you."

QUESTIONS FOR DISCUSSION

1. Should policies be flexible when handlers work alone or independently as part of a program? Are policies just guidelines?

2. How can handlers create opportunities to actively engage clients?

3. Should infractions such as the one experienced by Cindy be reported to the administration or program personnel from the therapy dog organization?

4. Should what happened to her dog Jack be reported as a safety violation or breach?

5. Did Cindy exercise poor judgement?

6. Should there be a change to policy to support handlers working independently with little on-site program support?

The featured scenario sets the stage for our discussion of policies, practices, and considerations when organizing and implementing canine-assisted interventions (CAIs). Addressing policies, practices, and considerations is important as they provide a structure to the program in which CAIs are offered, and most importantly, they help safeguard the welfare of all the different agents involved in a CAI – program personnel, handlers, therapy dogs, and clients. The aim of this chapter is to identify and elucidate policies and practices that optimize dog-handler team welfare. We begin with an examination of program design considerations or a priori program policies following which we turn our attention to the considerations within sessions and the practices therein that optimize dog and handler welfare. Our chapter concludes with a discussion of the gold standard practices upholding dog-handler welfare when conducting research.

WELFARE CONSIDERATIONS IN PROGRAM DESIGN

Embedding Welfare in the Organization's Mission/Vision Statement

To reflect the priority that dog-handler welfare holds within a therapy dog organization, issues of welfare should be embedded within the organization's mission or vision. This might take the form of a declarative statement regarding welfare (e.g., "Optimizing therapy dog welfare undergirds all our practices and informs our assessment protocols, the professional development of handlers, the scheduling of dog-handler teams, the duration of sessions, and the number of clients supported."), maybe reflected by a commitment to handler training (e.g., offering an educational session on the signs of canine stress), or through program personnel assigned to monitor welfare within sessions.

Rigorous Assessment of Dog-Handler Teams

Detailing assessment procedures to identify suitable dog-handler teams is beyond the scope of our book, and readers are directed to prior publications on this topic (e.g., Binfet & Hartwig, 2020) or to the websites of established therapy dog organizations to learn of different requirements for team selection (e.g., Pet Partners, n.d.). As we've discussed throughout this book, the rigorous assessment of handlers and their therapy dogs, both individually and collectively as a team, helps identify teams that are well suited to the demands of volunteering in CAIs. As we've previously noted, the careful screening, assessment, and evaluation of teams help ensure that the team is well positioned to withstand the stressors inherent in CAI participation – that is, that they develop and possess a certain *resiliency*. One aspect of the assessment of therapy dog-handler teams that optimizes team welfare is found in providing opportunity for the dogs to become familiar with, and practice, the skills they'll be tested on. That is, there should be ample transparency around the criteria being assessed and affording dogs the opportunity to become familiar with the testing environment, the personnel conducting the assessments, and the opportunity to practice the behaviours required as part of the assessment, collectively reflects protocols in support of dog welfare (Figure 7.2).

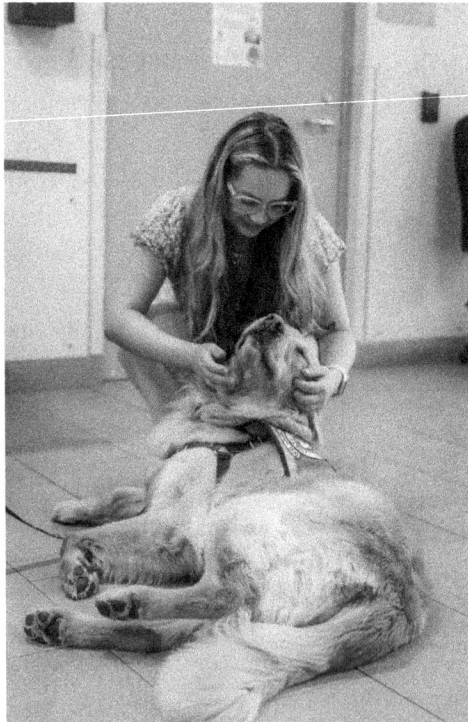

Figure 7.2 Therapy dog Abby lying down enjoying an interaction with a client who is gently stroking her face
Source: Freya L. L. Green Photography; used with permission

Extending our discussion in Chapter 5, our understanding of therapy dog welfare within the context of the assessment of dog-handler teams is also informed by review research by Miller and colleagues (2022) who argue for the need to not uniquely focus on what constitutes as unacceptable and indicators of unsuitability but rather focus on the indicators in therapy dogs that suggest they enjoy the tasks characterizing participation in a CAI – it is insufficient to focus solely on indicators of unsuitability or what constitutes as unacceptable. This innovative and refreshing perspective counters the focus on identifying reasons why therapy dogs are ill-suited to support clients and rather seeks to balance therapy dog assessments by considering and including factors or indicators reflecting that dogs are thriving and well suited for CAI work. In addition to biomarker indicators (i.e., cortisol, oxytocin), it is recommended that the assessment of therapy dogs include positive indicators such as providing opportunity for affective engagement between dogs and clients, identifying positive facial expressions in dogs as conveyed through ear movements and shifts in eye shape, and assessments of therapy dogs that incorporate the dog's positioning and movements. These researchers also raise the notion that play between dogs and clients should be invited and allows dogs to demonstrate behaviours reflecting positive engagement such as bowing and paw lifting. Miller and colleagues (2022) also raise the issue that different breeds may demonstrate such positive behaviours differently and that breeds such as Golden Retrievers and Labradors are characterized by greater displays of affection than other breeds (McCullough et al., 2018). As we've discussed in Chapter 5, personnel in therapy dog organizations responsible for the assessment of therapy dogs should be mindful of these breed differences (Figure 7.3).

Innovations in the formal assessment of therapy dogs have emerged, and we might see organizations leverage standardized measures to determine which dog-handler teams are best suited to the work they undertake. Take, for example, the *Canine Behaviour Assessment and Research Questionnaire* (CBARQ), a scale designed to rate dogs' temperament, trainability, and aggression (Hare et al., 2024; Sakurama et al., 2023). In other recent research, a systematic review of 3,891 publications and analysis of 39 studies by de Winkel and colleagues (2024) identified nine different behavioural categories or themes that afford assessors a window into dog behaviour and emotion – proxies for welfare.

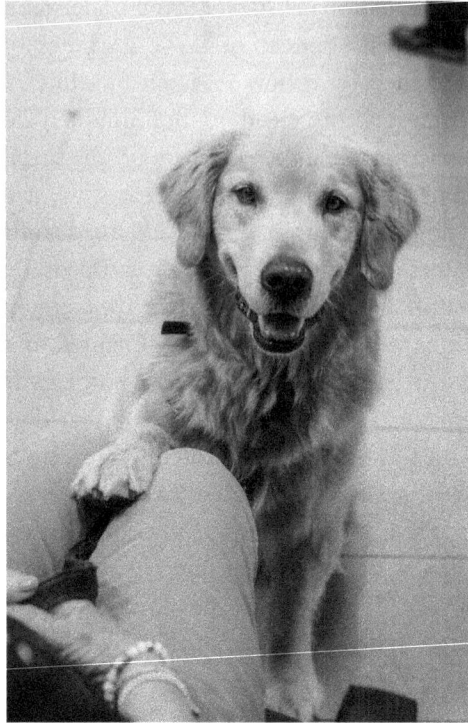

Figure 7.3 Therapy dog Doogle indicating additional interaction is welcomed as he smiles with his paw gently resting in someone's lap
Source: Freya L. L. Green Photography; used with permission

These include body posture, vocalizations, oral behaviour, observational physiological response to stress, other stress-related behaviours, interactions with non-social and social environments, emotional expressions, and the holistic observation of the dog's state. Collectively, the research described above holds potential to inform therapy dog organizations around how they might determine the suitability of dogs with strong consideration for dog welfare.

Incremental On-Boarding of New Teams

Once teams have been accepted for participation in a CAI, they should be incrementally on-boarded. That is, teams should not be immediately scheduled for participation in full sessions but rather scheduled for shortened visits to allow the team to become familiar with protocols and to build capacity and resiliency. In this regard, the on-boarding of teams helps safeguard dog-handler welfare by not overloading teams too quickly and allowing them to develop capacity over time. Doing so helps ensure that dogs, in particular, have repeated enjoyable experiences. Dogs should always leave sessions before their behaviour tells the handler that they're disengaged and done. As noted in the guidelines from the International Association of Human-Animal Interaction Organizations (IAHAIO, 2021, p. 3), "The time that animals spend interacting with clients, staff and visitors should be documented, and limited to the capacity of the individual animal."

Partnering with a Veterinarian

Partnering with a veterinarian offers a whole host of benefits for a therapy dog organization as there are dimensions or elements of coordinating interactions between therapy dogs and members of the public that are best informed by someone with advanced veterinary medical knowledge. Before we explore these benefits, it merits mention that just as there are benefits for the therapy dog organization arising from a partnership with a veterinarian, so too are there benefits that arise for the veterinarian. Most notably, this is seen in both the referral of new clients to the clinic and the frequency of visits by handlers seeking to maintain their dog's health in compliance with the requirements of the therapy dog organization under which they volunteer (e.g., routine fecal testing). Once established, the veterinarian and a technician can be invited to conduct a site visit and possibly observe a CAI session in action. This affords the veterinarian an opportunity to witness the nature of the interactions, the proximity of dogs to clients, the number of dogs working concurrently in the same space, the welfare mechanisms in place to support dogs, and the environmental conditions in which the dogs are asked to work.

Turning our attention now to the benefits for therapy dog organizations arising from partnering with a veterinarian, we first see a veterinarian helping guide the therapy dog organization in identifying the necessary health records to be documented for each dog-handler team. This might include vaccination records, submitting an annual health certificate, routine fecal testing, and information about the dog's diet (i.e., whether to allow a raw diet). Second, collaborating with a veterinarian can also assist a program in determining the minimum age of dogs to be considered for acceptance into programming. Here again, we see ample variation in recommendations around minimum age, recognizing that puppies are generally ill-equipped to deal with the demands placed on therapy dogs as part of a CAI. Further, puppies are generally considered to have less robust immune systems than older dogs and thus are considered more susceptible to becoming sick (Liguori et al., 2023; Meers et al., 2022). It has also been argued that puppies exige a more intimate or physically interactive interaction within a CAI that sees clients hold puppies or cuddle them close, and this, in turn, can facilitate zoonotic transmission (Meers et al., 2022). These precautions stated, we do see puppies occasionally participate in CAI research. In recent innovative research by Howell and colleagues (2024), nine puppies (ranging in age from 4 to 12 months) being raised as assistance dogs participated in a CAI to assess the effects of interactions on students' and staff members' stress and viality. The puppies participating in this research were a part of an established, on-campus initiative at La Trobe University called *Dogs for Life* where the monitoring of canine welfare is embedded within all care and initiatives involving the puppies. Here we see an example of a unique context that positions canine welfare front and centre in the puppies' rearing, training, and participation in research. Not touted as a benefit arising from their study, but undoubtedly, the puppies' participation in this study held potential benefits for the socialization of these future assistance dogs.

Third, consultation with a veterinarian can also help establish policy around requirements that potential dogs be spayed or neutered prior to acceptance into the program. Again, we see variability across programs; however, a scan of online program requirements suggests most programs requiring dogs to be spayed/neutered (Hartwig & Binfet, 2019). Fourth, collaborating with a veterinarian allows the therapy dog organization to understand and establish policy around retiring therapy dogs. Decisions around a therapy dog's retirement should be made in consultation with the dog's veterinarian, the handler, and the organization (including consideration of the demands of the programs in question) in order for an informed decision around retirement to occur. We recognize that older therapy dogs may bring a wealth of experience working in CAIs to sessions but that their capacity to withstand the stressors inherent in sessions (i.e., travel to and from sites, interacting with multiple clients, etc.)

can diminish over time. And last, partnering with a veterinarian can inform the therapy dog organization around best practices to reduce zoonotic transmission and the risk of infectious diseases. "Zoonotic infection can be transmitted both ways (human to animal, animal to human), and it is possible for both human and non-human animal participants within therapy dog programs to be at risk (Menna et al., 2019)" (McDowall et al., 2023, p. 6). To this latter point, additional information on reverse zoonosis or zooanthroponosis (i.e., the transmission of disease from humans to animals) can be found in recent work by Anderson and colleagues (2023) that elucidates reverse zoonotic transmission by explicating infections affecting both humans and animals.

In recent research by Boyle and colleagues (2019), it is argued that handlers' awareness and knowledge of the risks of zoonotic disease transmission and infectious diseases can help mitigate risks within the context of animal-assisted interventions (AAIs). For a review of zoonotic risks in AAIs readers are directed to recent research by Liguori and colleagues (2023) who have examined zoonosis and AAI from a One Health perspective. We have argued above that there are benefits for both therapy dog organizations and veterinarians in establishing a partnership. Importantly, we discussed numerous advantages for therapy dog organizations around the establishment of protocols for the assessment of dog-hander teams and around the implementation of CAIs. Certainly, one key advantage is that veterinarians can advise organizations around best practices to reduce both zoonosis and zooanthroponosis and, in this way, safeguard the welfare of both therapy dog-handler team and clients.

Training and Education for Handlers

Documentation for handlers is required too and should include a criminal record background check and emergency contact information. Regularly updated criminal record checks are required by some organizations as a means of helping ensure that handlers working with vulnerable populations are well suited to the task.

Beyond attending a "New Handler Orientation" session, ongoing professional development for handlers should be made available. This might include information regarding innovations in supporting clients served in the program (e.g., a professional development session on self-harm in college students for handlers volunteering in an on-campus CAI to support handlers when students disclose). Some programs may require annual recertification or credentialling involving updating and reviewing documentation for dogs and handlers and requiring the team to pass an abbreviated assessment to maintain good standing within the organization. Across organizations, there is ample variability around both the offering of professional development for handlers and the annual recredentialling of teams.

In addition to formal opportunities for handlers to engage in professional development, some programs may incorporate formative training within sessions as a way of supporting handler skill development. This might include program personnel offering feedback around leash tension entering or exiting a session, the positioning of dogs to foster client accessibility, or drawing the handler's attention to overlooked dog behavioural signs (e.g., that the dog is signaling that a break is needed). In this regard, this formative feedback is offered in-the-moment when it is likely to be most meaningful and relevant. Correspondingly, it goes without saying that handlers themselves must be open to this model and not bristle at suggestions to reconfigure or adjust their management of their dog. Handlers must see themselves like the feedback – in formation or constant evolution with regard to managing and advocating for their dog.

Establishing a Protocol for the Ratio of Clients to Each Dog-Handler Team

One policy that should be established a priori, especially in the light of the popularity of CAIs, is the ratio of clients to each dog-handler team. To avoid dogs being swarmed by overenthusiastic clients which can result in dogs not having a pathway to retreat from interactions, establishing the maximum number of clients per dog-handler station, helps safeguard both the dog and handler welfare. A ratio of three to four clients per dog, pending there is room for clients to interact comfortably, not crowd the dog, and leave the dog with a clear retreat pathway, would be considered the maximum number of clients per station. Consideration must be given too to handlers here as they interact with each client at their station and this, over time, can be taxing (Figure 7.4).

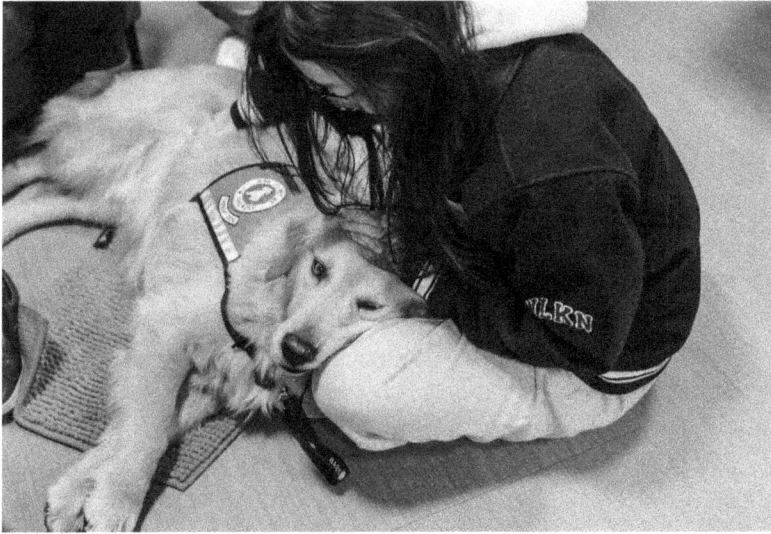

Figure 7.4 Doogle, an experienced therapy dog, leans against a client who gently rests her hand on his forehead
Source: Freya L. L. Green Photography; used with permission

Scheduling Dog-Handler Teams

Booking the optimal number of dog-handler teams helps safeguard dog-handler team welfare. Oftentimes the desire to interact with therapy dogs can surpass the therapy dog organization's capacity to meet this interest. Recall the scenario from Chapter 1 that saw a new volunteer handler Susan and her Golden Retriever Ollie participate in what she described as an on-campus "high-speed therapy dog factory." Here we saw the demand to interact with dog-handler teams surpass the organization's ability to support client interest. Restricting the number of clients served or increasing the number of available dog-handler teams must be considered to avoid overcrowding dogs and overwhelming handlers. On the flipside of this and as we saw in the scenario at the outset of this chapter, a handler volunteering by herself with no program personnel available found herself with no relief support to allow her a break in her role as a volunteer handler in a residential care facility program for seniors. Striking a balance in booking the right number of dogs to meet client and handler needs is key to the successful delivery of a CAI and ensuring optimal therapy dog welfare.

If the duration of interventions reported in research findings is any indication, there is ample variability in just how long therapy dog-handler teams are asked to participate in CAIs (see Table 7.1). Granted, oftentimes, the duration of a CAI is a variable intentionally manipulated by researchers (e.g., see recent research by Manville and colleagues (2023) assessing the effects of two-, five-, and ten-minute CAIs) but reflecting on the duration of a typical session is important for therapy dog organizations – especially with regard to safeguarding therapy dog welfare. Establishing a maximum session duration is key, and recommendations from the field suggest that 90 minutes is the upper limit for teams to be participating in sessions. Further, restrictions on the number of sessions per week should be established with teams not participating in more than two sessions in any given week (Table 7.1).

Table 7.1 Illustrations of Dose Intervention in Research

Study	Dose Intervention (min)	Number of Sessions per Week	Duration of Intervention (weeks)	Number of Participants
Barker et al. (2015)	10	1	1	40
Barker et al. (2016)	15	1	1	57
Binfet & Passmore (2016)	45	1	8	44
Chu et al.(2009)	50	1	8	30
Crossman & Kazdin (2015)	7 to 10	1	1	67
Fung & Leung (2014)	20	3	7	10
Grajfoner et al. (2016)	20	1	1	132
Havener et al. (2001)	-	1	1	40
Johnson et al. (2008)	15	3	4	30
Martin & Farnum (2002)	15	3	15	10
Schuck et al. (2015)	120-150	2	12	24
Vagnoli et al. (2015)	-	1	1	50
Villalta-Gil et al. (2009)	45	2	25	21

Note: - indicates data not reported.

Source: Binfet & Hartwig, 2020 in Anthrozoös; used with permission.

WELFARE CONSIDERATIONS IN PROGRAM DELIVERY – WITHIN-SESSION POLICIES

There are several practices that warrant consideration as program personnel offer CAIs to members of the public.

Therapy Dog Welfare as a Distributed Responsibility

It is not uniquely the program personnel's responsibility or the handler's responsibility to advocate for therapy dog welfare within sessions. Rather, this is a responsibility of everyone who designs, organizes, delivers, and attends a CAI.

Assigning Dog Welfare Monitor

Where resources permit, there should ideally be a representative from the therapy dog organization whose sole and unique task is to monitor therapy dog welfare. This person would have received prior training in canine behaviour with a particular emphasis on signs of canine stress/distress.

Handler Responsibility to Advocate for Therapy Dog Welfare

As part of their Handler Orientation or their new handler training protocols, handlers should be trained in recognizing signs of canine stress and discomfort. Handlers are uniquely positioned to recognize shifts in their dog's behaviour and to make adjustments to reduce stimuli (e.g., repositioning a dog so reduce distractions from other dog-handler teams) or to implement a break to allow the dog to recalibrate or toilet. Handlers must prioritize their dog's welfare and not feel pressure to persist within a session out of fear of disappointing program personnel or a line of clients eagerly awaiting admission to the session.

Graphic Aids as Reminders That Dog Welfare Is a Priority

In addition to delegating responsibility to program personnel to monitor therapy dog welfare within sessions and ensuring that handlers are trained in recognizing signs of canine stress, some programs make use of graphic aids to remind all agents of their duty to be vigilant in safeguarding welfare (see Appendix 7.1). Such reminders serve to raise awareness of the importance of canine welfare and of the distributed responsibility of everyone who partakes in a CAI to play a role in upholding welfare protocols.

Allowing Time for Dogs to Settle

Upon arrival to the space where the CAI will be offered, dog-handler teams require time to settle, dogs in particular. As discussed in Chapter 5, there are a number of stimuli to which dogs must adjust including adapting to the flooring, odours, and possibly working in close proximity to other dog-handler teams. Providing dogs have been toileted and, pending their prior experience, we have seen dogs take five to seven minutes to comfortably settle at their station and longer even for dogs who are in the process of on-boarding and who are still building their capacity to work in CAIs. As discussed previously, dogs who fail to settle (i.e., continue to pace or explore) may need an additional toilet break or it could be that they are ill-equipped to participate in the session with the team being sent home (Figure 7.5).

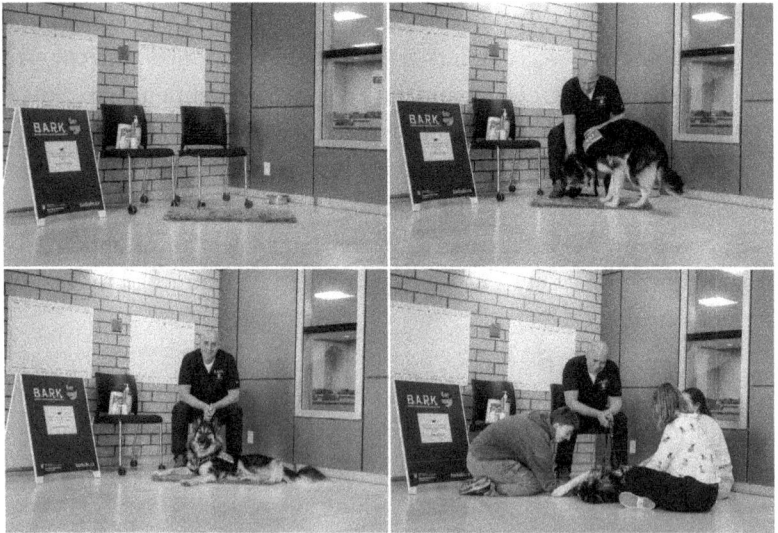

Figure 7.5 Series demonstrating handler John-Tyler inviting his therapy dog Henry to their assigned station, allowing time for Henry to settle into new working space before welcoming clients

Source: Freya L. L. Green Photography; used with permission

Water Bowls and Comfort Mats

As dog-handler teams may be scheduled for sessions up to 90 minutes, a reasonable expectation is that each station is equipped with water for the dog and the handler, a comfort mat for the dog, and comfortable seating for handlers. Collectively, these considerations help optimize the dog-handler team welfare and ensure they are well positioned to supporting clients.

Dog Under Handler Control and Supervision at All Times

Regardless of whether there are program personnel available to help monitor dog welfare, therapy dogs working as part of CAIs are to remain under the vigilant supervision of their handlers. It is not uncommon for clients to challenge this model and ask to walk dogs or to connect more directly with dogs beyond the scope of the inter-action typically afforded within a CAI. In on-campus CAIs, we might see a university student ask a handler, "My friends are studying outside in the hall, can I take him out to show them?" Here an invitational redirection by the handler works best to acknowledge the enthusiasm of the student while respecting program policy for the supervision of dogs (Figure 7.6). A handler in this case might respond, "We can't do that but your friends are welcome to visit us here."

Limited Inter-dog Socialization

We've previously addressed the notion of dog socialization, and to encourage dogs to be client-focused, we recommend limited inter-dog interaction. As we noted, there are times when dogs have established friendships with other dogs, and we have found allowing these dogs a quick hello goes a long way in helping them settle at their stations. Some handlers might have the notion that volunteering on behalf of a therapy dog organization is a good way to socialize dogs. Certainly, we have found that dogs become socialized to working in public spaces and to interacting with varied members of the public, but in an effort to reduce the possibility of any inter-dog conflict, we recommend limiting dogs interacting with other dogs.

No Client Food in Sessions

As we saw in our opening scenario, food can tempt even the most well-trained dog. Recall the incident where Jack, a therapy dog working in a retirement facility in support of senior residents was led

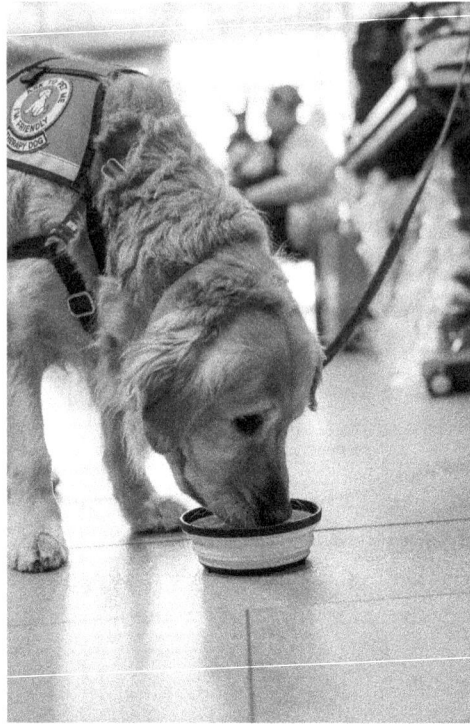

Figure 7.6 Therapy dog Dash enjoys a break to drink water from her own bowl while participating in a CAI

Source: Freya L. L. Green Photography; used with permission

through the cafeteria by a resident and fed treats. A clear policy that no food (dog treats nor human food brought in by clients) is allowed in sessions. Doing so helps reduce temptation for dogs and helps optimize their ability to focus on the clients at their station.

Handler Determines the End of Session in Collaboration with Program Personnel

As we've argued previously, the session should be terminated BEFORE the dog signals that they have had enough and are no longer interested in participating. That is, the dog's participation in a session should be curtailed prior to the dog exhausting their ability to continue participating. Again, the handler is at the helm of the decision-making surrounding the ending of a session and, in consultation with program personnel (if available), should determine when their dog should

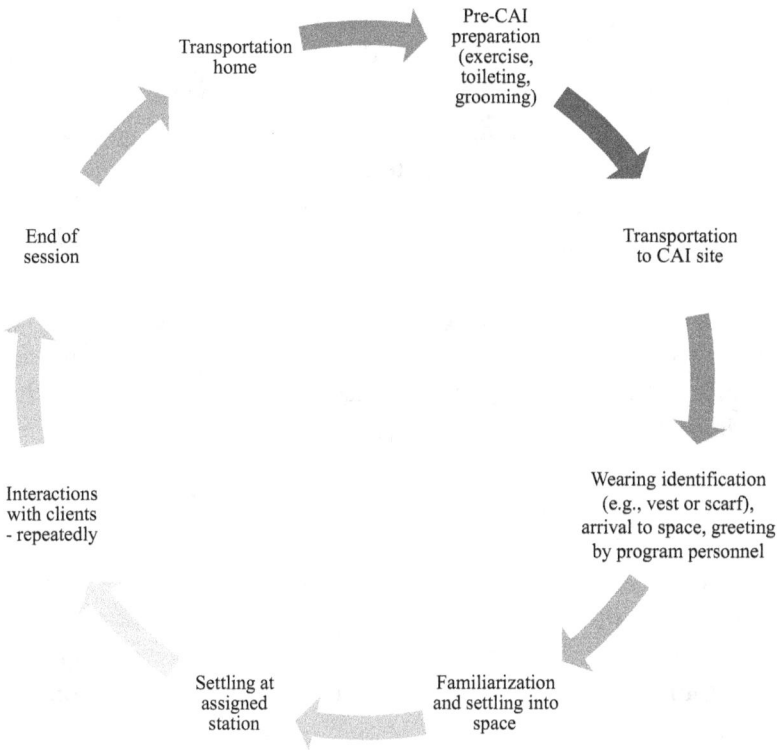

Figure 7.7 Choreography of participating in a CAI

leave – even if before the end of their scheduled session. Welfare takes priority over scheduling.

Recognizing the Dynamic Nature of a Session

There is a certain choreography that occurs for dog-handler teams participating in CAIs, and we recognize that there are different stages of a CAI which might include those shown in Figure 7.7.

GOLD STANDARD RESEARCH PRACTICES THAT OPTIMIZE WELFARE

There are a number of practices that can be implemented to optimize welfare within CAI research. First, when designing methodologies where the CAI constitutes the independent variable, researchers are to consult and cite prior research to discern what's been previously done by other CAI researchers and why. That is, unless replicating a study, researchers are to build upon prior methodology. This might include identifying the duration of the intervention (e.g., abbreviated or at the determination of participants), the mode of delivery of the CAI (e.g., in person, virtually), the number of participants supported by each dog-handler team (i.e., the ratio of handler and dog to participants), whether handlers follow a script or reference a bank of questions to engage participants, and whether the CAI itself required any particular modification or manipulation (e.g., requiring participants to touch or not touch dogs). This is not to say that researchers cannot forge new empirical territory by introducing creative or novel new approaches. Rather, we're arguing here that methodologies and procedures should acknowledge past research and build upon it.

Second, as should be standard practice, both animal and human research ethics' applications must be submitted. Doing so allows an external body to review study procedures and ensure no harm is caused to any of the study participants – be they humans participating in the intervention or therapy dogs who are a key component of the intervention. Submission of an animal research ethics application will require researchers to disclose the training or credentialling of therapy dogs, the number of dogs participating, the duration of their participation, the circumstances of their participation including under whose supervision the dogs will be, and any particular activities the dogs might be asked to do.

Third, researchers must report whether any a priori training of the dog-handler teams was implemented. As discussed previously, such might be the case when CAIs are implemented within specialized contexts or with unique populations (think individuals who are incarcerated within a detention centre or perhaps police members within a busy detachment). Training for dog-handler teams might include a review of safety protocols or familiarization with the research environment prior to the study. Familiarization with study protocols and the space or location of the study help therapy dogs settle and reduce the chance of dogs being ill at ease on the day of data collection.

Fourth, as part of the measures administered, demographic information regarding both the handler and the therapy dog should be collected. This might include asking handlers to report their and their dog's age, their gender, and the extent of their prior experience volunteering as part of CAIs. Capturing this information allows researchers to report information describing the agents delivering the intervention. Consider for a moment how an intervention that sees new volunteer handlers and their dogs participate in an intervention might be different from the same intervention delivered by experienced dog-handler teams. As we argued and illustrated in Chapter 1, the experience of the team adds value to the intervention and increases the likelihood that the intervention will have uptake and that outcome variables will be impacted.

Fifth, steps must be taken prior to the start of the study to safeguard therapy dog welfare. This might include ensuring the temperature in the room is optimal for dogs and runs cool rather than warm/hot and the experimental space has been cleaned so as to ensure dogs avoid dropped food, medication, or harmful objects such as tacks or staples; creating stations or identifying space for each dog-handler team and ensuring there is sufficient distance separating dog-handler teams from other teams; providing a comfort mat and water bowl for dogs; and having someone in the room whose sole task is to oversee and monitor dog welfare. Also included in these protocols is a provision for dogs who fail to settle, who appear agitated, or who indicate they'd like to leave the session or refuse to participate in the CAI. Oftentimes, a toileting break is offered to dogs to see if that alleviates this unease allowing them to return to the study after their break. Should the dog continue to be unsettled, the dog-handler team is sent home. Researchers should plan to have substitute dog-handler teams on standby in the event a team must be replaced. Should any dog-handler team withdraw from the study, researchers should report this as it is one reflection of implementation fidelity.

Sixth, researchers must report whether there are any breaches of safety occurred as a part of the study and describe the nature of these and any action taken. This might include a dog who was fearful of a participant and retreated, thus compromising the delivery of the intervention or any participant behaviour that threatened dog welfare requiring research personnel to take action (e.g., a participant who fails to follow study procedures).

Next, researchers using CAIs as the independent variable in their study must consider the length of time it takes participants to complete measures vis-à-vis the duration of the intervention. Oftentimes we see researchers experiment with abbreviated durations as we did in our Virtual Canine Comfort study described in Chapter 6. As the intervention was but five minutes, it would be hard to justify having participants complete a battery of measures taking 20–30 minutes to complete. We argue that the best practice is for researchers to align the time it takes participants to complete self-report measures with the duration of the intervention itself. With abbreviated intervention durations, we often see researchers employ one-item or Visual Analogue Scales to measure outcome variables (e.g., stress, loneliness, etc.).

And last, researchers are not to be involved as handlers in their own study and with their own personal dog and should collaborate with credentialled dog-handler teams. We mentioned in Chapter 4 that accessing therapy dog-handler teams can be challenging, and we've seen research where the researcher themself served in the dual role as a researcher and as a handler delivering the intervention. Doing so is complicated for a number of reasons. First, that the researcher is serving as a handler in their own study and serving in a dual capacity, and should be disclosed as part of both the human and animal ethics' applications. Second, when the researcher serves as a handler in their own study, they have a vested interest in the intervention working as it was hypothesized or intended. This introduces unnecessary biases and may call into question the integrity of the intervention, thereby compromising study results. Last, given the vested interest from the researcher that the study plays out as planned, they may be poorly positioned to monitor their dog's welfare. Collectively, the above reasons, and likely others, argue against researchers serving in dual capacities as both the experimenter and the handler.

CONCLUSION

The aim of this chapter was to explore factors within the design of therapy dog programs and the delivery of sessions within these programs that optimize dog-handler team welfare. We examined design characteristics such as assessing dog-handler teams with consideration of their capacity to develop resiliency and, relatedly, the slow on-boarding of teams into programs to safeguard dog welfare and help dogs develop the capacity to withstand the stressors inherent in a CAI session. We also explored factors within sessions optimizing dog-handler team welfare such as allowing dogs to settle into spaces before the arrival of clients, not allowing clients to bring food into sessions, and providing water and a comfort mat for dogs. We raised the issue as well of assigning personnel to monitor therapy dog welfare and to convey to all agents that dog welfare is a shared and distributed responsibility – borne by program personnel, handlers, and the clients who make use of CAIs. We concluded this chapter with a series of recommendations for researchers conducting CAI research and outlined the steps they might take to safeguard dog-handler team welfare. In our next and last chapter that follows, we synthesize key concepts raised within previous chapters and cast an eye to future directions.

REFERENCES

Anderson, B. D., Barnes, A. N., Umar, S., Guo, X., Thongthum, T., & Gray, G. C. (2023). Reverse zoonotic transmission (Zooanthroponosis): An increasing threat to animal health. In A. Sing (Ed.), *Zoonoses: Infections affecting humans and animals* (pp. 1–63). Springer.

Binfet, J. T., & Hartwig, E. K. (2020). *Canine-assisted interventions: A comprehensive guide to credentialing therapy dog teams*. Routledge.

Boyle, S. F., Corrigan, V. K., Buechner-Maxwell, V., & Pierce, B. J. (2019). Evaluation of risk of zoonotic pathogen transmission in a university-based animal assisted intervention (AAI) program. *Frontiers in Veterinary Science, 6*, Article 167. https://doi.org/10.3389/fvets.2019.00167

de Winkel, T., van der Steen, S., Enders-Slegers, M. J., Giffioen, R., Haverbeke, A., Groenewoud, D., & Hediger, K. (2024). Observationsl behaviors and emotions to assess welfare in dogs: A systematic review. *Journal of Veterinary Behavior, 72*, 1–17. https://doi.org/10.1016/j.jveb.2023.12.007

Hare, E., Essler, J. L., Otto, C. M., Ebbecke, D., & Serpell, J. A. (2024). Development of a modified C-BARQ for evaluating behavior in working dogs. *Frontiers in Veterinary Science, 11*, 1371630. https://doi.org/10.3389/fvets.2024.1371630

Hartwig, E., & Binfet, J. T. (2019). What's important in canine-assisted intervention teams? An investigation of canine-assisted intervention program online screening tools. *Journal of Veterinary Behavior: Clinical Applications and Research, 29*, 53–60. https://doi.org/10.1016/j.jveb.2018.09.004

Howell, T. J., Mai, D. L., Dragonovic, P., Binfet, J. T., & Bennett, P. C. (2024). Impact of interactions with a puppy and handler versus a handler alone on stress and vitality in a university setting: A crossover study. *ANIMALS, 14*, 2454. https://doi.org/10.3390/ani14172454

IAHAIO (2021). IAHAIO international guidelines on care, training and welfare requirements for small animals in animal-assisted interventions. Retrieved June 12, 2024 from: https://iahaio.org/wp/wp-content/uploads/2021/09/for-publication-small-animal-care-and-welfare-in-aai.pdf

Liguori, G., Costagliola, A., Lombardi, R., Paciello, O., & Giordano, A. (2023). Human-animal interaction in animal-assisted interventions (AAIs): Zoonosis risks, benefits, and future directions: A one health approach. *Animals*, 13, 1592. https://doi.org/10.3390/ani13101592

Manville, K., Coulson, M., & Reynolds, G. (2023). An exploratory randomised controlled trial comparing the effectiveness of different duration of canine-assisted interventions in high education students. *Human-Animal Interactions*, 11(1), https://doi.org/10.1079/hai.2023.0038

McCullough, A., Jenkins, M. A., Ruehrdanz, A., Gilmer, J. J., Olson, J.,... O'Haire, M. (2018). Physiological and behavioral effects of animal-assisted interventions on therapy dogs in pediatric oncology settings. *Applied Animal Behaviour Science*, 200, 86–95. https://doi.org/10.1016/j.applanim.2017.11.014

McDowall, S., Hazel, S. J., Cobb, M., & Hamilton-Bryce, A. (2023). Understanding the roleof therapy dogs in human health promotion. *International Journal of Environmental Research and Public Health*, 20, 5801. https://doi.org/10.3390/ijerph20105801

Meers, L. L., Contalbrio, L., Samuels, W. E., Duarte-Gan, C., Berckmans, D.,... Normando, S. (2022). Canine-assisted interventions and the relevance of welfare assessments for human health, and transmission of zoonosis: A literature review. *Frontiers in Veterinary Science*, 9, 899889. https://doi.org/10.3389/fvets.2022.899889

Menna, L., Santaniello, A., Todisco, M., Amato, A., Borrelli, L., Scandurra, C., & Fioretti. A. (2019). The human-animal relationship as the focus of animal-assisted interventions: A One Health approach. *International Journal of Environmental Research and Public Health*, 16, 3660. https://doi.org/10.3390/ijerph16193660

Miller, S. L., Serpell, J. A., Dalton, K. R., Waite, K. B., Morris, D. O.,... Davis, M. F. (2022). The importance of evaluating positive welfare characteristics and temperament in working therapy dogs. *Frontiers in Veterinary Sciences*, 4(9), 844252. https://doi.org/10.3389/fvets.2022.844252

Pet Partners (n.d.). *Program requirements.* Retrieved June 12, 2024 from: https://petpartners.org/volunteer/requirements/

Sakurama, M., Ito, M., Nakanowataru, Y., & Kooriyama, T. (2023). Selection of appropriate dogs to be therapy dogs using the C-BARQ. *Animals*, 13(5), 834–844. https://doi.org/10.3390/ani13050834

APPENDIX 7.1

Graphic Aid as a Reminder to Monitor Therapy Dog Welfare in Sessions
(Source: Building Academic Retention through K9s; used with permission)

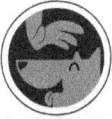 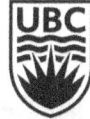

RECOGNIZING SIGNS OF K9 STRESS

PANTING
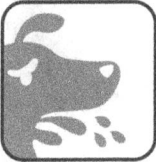

TURNING AWAY
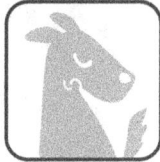

PAWING
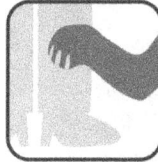

WHIMPERING
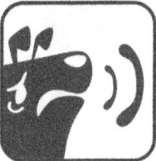

TREMBLING
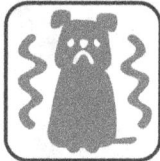

YAWNING
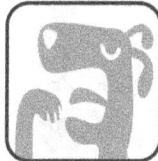

PACING
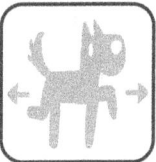

CHANGES IN BEHAVIOUR

After all, don't you act differently when you're stressed?

barkubc.ca   BARK UBCO   barkubc

Eight

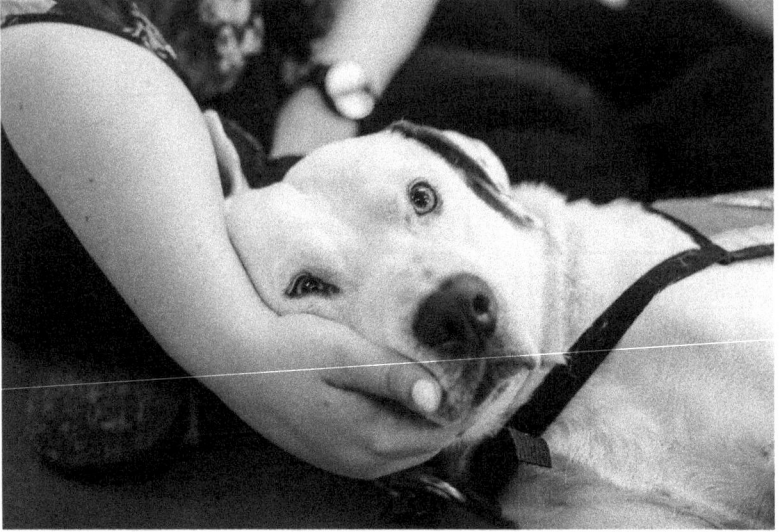

Figure 8.1 Therapy dog Dewey relaxes into a client's hand
Source: Freya L. L. Green Photography; used with permission

DOI: 10.4324/9781032639284-8

SCENARIO

She's Sick So I'm Stepping In

It was clear that Golden Retriever Chloe had been groomed and care and attention had been put into preparing her for today's on-campus stress reduction session. Led by a young man, who himself looked like a college student, Chloe appeared at ease and responded to commands given, sitting promptly at the entrance to the room as the young man checked in. "My mom is sick today so I'm stepping in. Which station is ours?" said the young man, introducing himself as Rich. Taken aback, and without any prior notification, the program director was struck by this sudden switch in handlers. On the one hand, she respected the handler's commitment to contribute despite being ill, but on the other hand, the replacement substitute had no knowledge of the policies and practices expected of handlers. Added to this, he seemed far too young himself to serve as a source of support for students his age who might be struggling with their stress management. Would he even be taken seriously? In need of dog-handler teams for the session and expecting robust attendance from students on campus, the program director felt torn and pulled in two directions (Figure 8.1).

QUESTIONS FOR DISCUSSION

1. Should a replacement handler familiar to the therapy dog be allowed?

2. What protocols should be established for a handler missing a session?

3. How might the therapy dog's welfare be compromised by a handler with no training and unfamiliar with program protocols?

4. Do handlers have skills above and beyond regular dog owners?

The featured scenario illustrates some of the complexities in offering canine-assisted intervention (CAI) programming in the face of high demand by clients and the realities that, at the heart of the programs, are volunteer handlers who have commitments beyond those to the therapy dog organization and who occasionally must miss sessions. Designing and delivering CAIs is no small undertaking and challenges are certain to arise. The aim of this last chapter is to unite key concepts introduced throughout our book and to cast an eye to the future. We consider here, what future directions practitioners and researchers might consider in offering and researching issues germane to CAIs?

SCENARIOS ILLUSTRATING THE COMPLEXITIES OF, AND CHALLENGES IN, CAI PROGRAMMING AND RESEARCH

As university professors teaching and researching in the fields of human-animal interactions (HAIs) and Animal-Assisted Interventions (AAIs), we recognize the need for realistic and challenging illustrations of CAIs. As such, we knew it important to offer scenarios for readers to provoke their thinking around how to safeguard and optimize dog-handler team welfare in real-world contexts – busy contexts where multiple agents with different interests or agendas might interact and potentially clash. In each scenario, and drawing from our applied experience, we positioned dog-handler teams in situations mirroring challenges we'd witnessed or tried to resolve ourselves. As you've seen, these challenges ran the gamut from a dog-handler team overwhelmed and under-supported at an on-campus stress reduction CAI to a scenario that saw a therapy dog fed French fries at an airport, to a situation in which a handler needing to use the restroom called into question policies at a residential care facility. Inherent in each of these scenarios are themes of therapy dog (and oftentimes handler) well-being.

Instructors teaching courses on HAI and AAI are invited to use these scenarios to clarify their own positioning around welfare and to, in turn, challenge and foster the critical thinking of their students in considering how to optimize welfare for therapy dogs and their handlers. Across the eight scenarios contained within this book and presented at the outset of each chapter, we hope to illustrate the complexities or "muddiness" in offering CAI programming or conducting CAI research. We hope too that these same scenarios will prove useful to therapy dog organizations as they reflect on how best to screen, assess, and select dog-handler teams that will uphold their organization's mission and vision. We foresee our scenarios as useful in helping prospective, and veteran handlers consider both their own practices and optimal practices as they participate in CAIs in varied contexts (Figure 8.2).

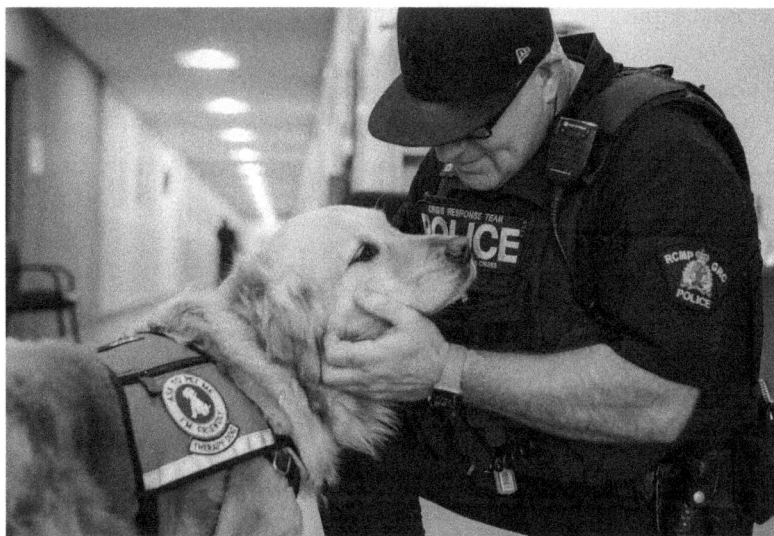

Figure 8.2 A police member wearing his uniform and radio interacts with therapy dog Abby as part of a CAI at an urban police detachment
Source: Freya L. L. Green Photography; used with permission

UNITING CONCEPTS ACROSS CHAPTERS

Our first chapter (Chapter 1) introduced readers to and defined CAIs – the catalyst or framework in which members of the public are afforded the opportunity to interact with therapy dogs in pursuit of one or several desired outcomes. This might include the reduction of stress or loneliness or to increase social interactions and build a sense of community among attendees. Therapy dog-handler teams, in this regard, are versatile, and we saw evidence, throughout this book, of how dog-handler teams participated in CAIs situated in schools, universities, public libraries, police detachments, and prison settings, among others. Also found in Chapter 1 was a clarification of terminology used in the broader field of AAIs, and we set the stage in this chapter for a discussion of dog-handler team *welfare*.

Our second chapter (Chapter 2) provided a historical overview of CAIs and their development over time. Herein we saw how pioneers in the fields of HAIs and AAIs laid the foundation for the innovative current CAI applied programming and research done today. A cornerstone of this chapter was the overview provided of the theoretical frameworks undergirding CAI programming and research. Here we saw biophilia, biopsychosocial, attachment, and social support theories explicated. This chapter concluded with a summary of the self-report and biomarker indicators attesting to the efficacy of CAIs as a modality bolstering human well-being.

Building upon the definition of welfare identified in Chapter 1, Chapter 3 saw us proffer a definition of therapy dog welfare unique and germane to therapy dogs working in CAIs. In Chapter 3, we defined therapy dog welfare as:

> Therapy dog welfare within a canine-assisted intervention is a state of well-being monitored and facilitated by a handler that sees the dog consent to an interaction with a human, demonstrate behaviours reflecting that the interaction is welcomed (e.g., prompting the human for additional petting, leaning into client, etc.), demonstrates behaviour free of agitation or distress (i.e., excessive panting, shaking, whale eye, etc.), and where the dog has the freedom to retreat from the interaction of their own freewill (i.e., not crowded and with a pathway to retreat) without negative consequences (i.e., redirection or correction from handler).

Embedded within this definition, we see themes of handler advocacy and responsibility, an emphasis on observable canine behavioural and emotional indicators of agency, enjoyment, and well-being reflecting the dog's willingness to consent to or retreat from interactions. Our intention in offering a definition of welfare specific to CAIs is that others will consider, refine, and determine the utility of this definition vis-à-vis supporting therapy dogs in the work they undertake. Also found within this chapter was consideration of handler well-being, an oft-overlooked dimension of welfare within CAIs. As part of this discussion of handler well-being, we introduced the notion of emotional contagion between handlers and dogs, a concept we explored subsequently in Chapter 5.

As part of Chapter 4, we examined pathways to accessing therapy dog-handler teams and elucidated the two dominant options of outsourcing teams and/or creating accessible teams through in-house program development. Accessing dog-handler teams for participation in varied events in support of varied clients remains a distinct challenge facing the field of CAIs, especially in the light of the increasing demand from the public to interact with therapy dogs. Next, we examined the individual and collective dispositions and skills required of both therapy dogs and handlers. A key theme we identified was the dog's genuine interest in, and curiosity to engage with, the public.

As part of Chapter 5, we examined factors fostering and impeding or compromising dog-handler team welfare and provided an overview of signs of both dog and handler stress. We highlighted the importance of and need for canine consent and revisited the notion of emotional contagion introduced in Chapter 3. Our chapter concluded with a Welfare Checklist, capturing for practitioners and researchers key considerations in safeguarding and optimizing dog-handler team welfare.

As we see both the interest in and demand for CAIs increase, expand, and diversify, Chapter 6 provided an overview of varied contexts and clients supported by CAIs. Here we examined and considered CAIs in school, post-secondary, medical, correctional facilities and virtual contexts, and highlighted the need for a nuanced assessment of dog-handler teams for work within these diverse settings. Chapter 6 concluded with a discussion of dog-handler teams supporting diverse and unique client populations.

Building upon the definition of welfare proposed in Chapter 3, Chapter 7 explored how welfare could be optimized through the design and delivery of CAI programming. Here we explored a priori considerations in the design of programs that included considerations of the assessment of dog-hander teams comprised of individual and collective assessments of dogs and handlers; the gradated on-boarding of teams to build capacity and resiliency, offering ongoing professional development to handlers; the frequency of scheduling dog-handler teams and the maximum duration of participation with a session; and consideration of the total number of clients supported within a session by a team. From an applied perspective, we offered recommendations to optimize dog-handler team welfare that included providing teams with water and a comfort mat, assigning personnel where possible to monitor welfare within sessions, and fostering a shared responsibility for therapy dog welfare across all agents – program personnel, handlers, and visiting clients. Our chapter concluded with a series of recommendations for researchers to consider as they honor therapy dog-handler team welfare as a core tenet of the work they undertake.

FUTURE DIRECTIONS

It was our intention throughout this book to raise awareness and discussion around the importance of safeguarding and optimizing therapy dog-handler team welfare. As we've argued, doing so ensures conditions are created in which both the dog and the handler can thrive and support the clients who make use of this popular well-being resource. From a theoretical perspective, our focus on optimizing therapy dog-handler team welfare aligns with new and inspiring ways of thinking about animals and HAIs that embrace a *One Health and Wellness* approach (Chalmers & Dell, 2015; Peralta & Fine, 2021; Pinillos, 2018) or *relational ontology* (Haraway, 2008; Shapiro, 2020) and seek to challenge traditional boundaries between humans and animals. As discussed in Chapter 2, these approaches recognize the interconnections between human welfare and animal welfare and call for a repositioning of therapy dogs, one that highlights reciprocity in therapy dogs' interactions with humans and is consistent with an ever-increasing focus on animal agency, enjoyment, and welfare in the context of CAIs (and AAIs; Ng et al., 2015). We've embraced and extended these ideas throughout this book, and we've positioned therapy dogs and handlers as a "cohesive team" whose positive contribution to human health and well-being is optimized when both therapy dog and handler welfare are prioritized.

From an applied perspective, CAIs are a low-cost and low-barrier resource with varied applicability – clients typically do not need to sign up for appointments to interact with dog-handler teams, and teams can be found working in a variety of settings in support of a variety of clients. From a research perspective, implementing welfare measures within methodological frameworks enhances the robustness of the intervention and increases implementation fidelity (i.e., reporting duration of sessions, the ratio of dog to clients, etc.; Rodriguez et al., 2023). A scan of CAI research reveals ample variability in how researchers situate and position CAIs as the independent variable eliciting change in a host of outcome variables – for dogs and human alike. A recent example of innovative research that positioned welfare as central to an on-campus CAI is found in the work of Williams and colleagues (2024) who co-constructed a *Paws on Campus* program to support student mental health. In consultation with student well-being representatives, veterinarians, animal welfare charities, and representatives from a therapy dog organization, these researchers "co-produced" an intervention comprised of four parts: (1) thoughts and feelings; (2) well-being and welfare; (3) care and compassion; and (4) problem-solving and help-seeking (see Williams et al., 2024 here). We suspect that this research will lay the foundation for additional research that sees researchers co-construct different iterations of CAIs to support well-being.

As we forecast trends in CAI-related research, we anticipate additional research assessing biomarker indicators of therapy dog well-being and an increased interest in the impact of participating in sessions on dog-handler teams. Do teams, as we've posited in our book, build capacity and resiliency over time or does participation in session, where exposure to clients often characterized by heightened levels of stress and/or loneliness, take a collective toll on teams, reducing their efficacy? Additional research investigating the impact of CAI participation on the well-being of teams is likely.

Related to the above and recall from Chapter 2 our review of research on touch, recent research has examined the mechanisms within interactions that contribute to well-being outcomes in human participants, especially around the role of touch (see Beetz, 2011; Binfet et al., 2022; Pendry & Vandagriff, 2019). As argued by Fournier (2019), Wagner and colleagues (2022), and others, despite the popularity of AAIs, we know little about the mechanisms that occur during HAIs that contribute to changes in outcome variables. Findings, to date, collectively suggest that touch may be key to optimizing well-being outcomes in humans, however no research has examined the impact of this touch on therapy dogs. Consider for a moment, just how many clients a therapy dog might support in each session and the amount of touch (i.e., petting, caressing) the dogs would experience. Although researchers suggest touch is beneficial for the humans participating in a CAI, what is the impact of touch on therapy dogs? Can there be too much touch? Might ambient proximity to therapy dogs suffice?

Related to the issue of touch within sessions, researchers should examine if a calm versus playful CAI differentially impacts client outcomes. As we discussed in Chapter 5, some therapy dogs might prefer interactive and playful versus calming interactions. We also saw in Chapter 6 how virtual contexts might be appealing to some clients and therapy dogs. For some therapy dogs, virtual interactions might reduce overwork and stress since there is no direct contact or hands-on interactions between the dog and the client and. In this way, virtual contexts might be ideal for optimizing welfare for therapy dogs who do not enjoy participating in CAIs. Research is needed to carefully examine the quality of interactions between varied clients and therapy dogs across multiple contexts to better understand the characteristics and conditions defining successful CAIs.

Also related to the above yet from the perspective of handlers, what might be the impact of handlers supporting multiple clients with heightened stress and/or loneliness? Is there a lingering effect on handler well-being from all of the interactions they experience? Handlers in general are an understudied component of CAIs, and future research might explore this aspect of handler well-being. Extending this further, we raised in Chapters 3 and 5 the notion of emotional contagion between dogs and handlers, and future research might examine whether emotional contagion or the passing of feelings of stress and loneliness from clients to handlers occurs.

Stepping back from the need for research on the effects of a CAI on handlers themselves, there is a pressing need to understand how best to recruit handlers for participation in CAI programming and research. This issue was highlighted in Chapter 3 when we showcased research by Eaton-Stull and colleagues (2023) who conducted surveys of handlers volunteering within the context of animal-assisted crisis response (AACR). These researchers argued that "maintaining qualified volunteers is challenging" (p. 1). This aligns with the discourse throughout our book that positions the desire to interact with therapy dogs by varied members of the public surpassing the capabilities of dog-therapy organizations to provide access to dog-handler teams to meet this need. Additional research is needed to understand the motivations of handlers to elucidate the reasons drawing them to, and keeping them volunteering in, CAI programming. Doing so holds potential to inform dog-handler team recruitment efforts. There are research implications arising from the challenge in finding qualified dog-handler teams too. Above and beyond the question of accessing teams, might dog-handler teams participating in research initiatives be held to higher qualification expectations than those participating uniquely in applied programming?

We established in Chapter 1 that there has been exponential growth in AAI and CAI research. This is evidenced by the sheer volume of publications devoted to understanding HAI, AAI, CAI, and the human-animal bond. There is certainly keen interest in all things "therapy dogs," and throughout our book, we explored and showcased therapy dogs working in a variety of settings ranging from school classrooms to university classrooms and from public libraries to detention centres. Recent news coverage of a therapy dog titled "A day in the life of Beacon, the therapy dogs at US Olympic gymnastics trials" (ESPN, 2024) extends the sphere of settings in which therapy dogs have been found and raises questions around the practice of having therapy dogs in such contexts, notably around dog welfare. Future research might assess the suitability of contexts to support the integration of CAIs and dog-handler teams. What characterizes a context in which dog-handler teams might thrive?

Welfare Audits?

As we conclude our book, we leave readers with a provocation – Might *Welfare Audits* for therapy dog organizations be a useful means through which the welfare of dog-handler teams can be determined? Conducted by an independent governing body, might organizations receive a review and a corresponding rating reflecting the extent to which dog-handler team welfare is honored, protected, and upheld? What might this process look like? What criteria might be used to determine low-, medium-, or high-quality welfare practices? Would organizations find this process useful? Would clients seeking to interact with therapy dogs reference audit outcomes in choosing a therapy dog organization with which to partner?

CONCLUSION

Our hope in writing this book was to respond to the need for increased information and discussion about therapy dog-handler welfare within the context of CAIs. We've drawn both on prior research and from our applied practice and experience in designing and offering CAIs to varied client populations across varied contexts. We strove throughout our book to honour dog welfare – to advocate for, identify, and recommend practices that help create optimal conditions in which dogs, under the advocacy and guidance of their handlers, can engage with and support clients, enjoy their interactions, and contribute to the promotion of human well-being. We hope readers can leverage information found throughout this book as they design and implement CAI programming or conduct research exploring and examining varied aspects of CAIs.

REFERENCES

Beetz, A., Kotrschal, K., Turner, D. C., Hediger, K., Uvnäs-Moberg, K., & Julius, H. (2011). The effect of a real dog, toy dog and friendly person on insecurely attached children during a stressful task: An exploratory study. *Anthrozoös*, 24(4), 349–368. https://doi.org/10.2752/175303711X13159027359746

Binfet, J. T., Green, F. L. L., & Draper, Z. A. (2022). The importance of client-canine contact in canine-assisted interventions: A randomized controlled trial. *Anthrozoös*, 35(1), 1–22. https://doi.org/10.1080/08927936.2021.1944558

Chalmers, D., & Dell, C. A. (2015). Applying one health to the study of animal-assisted interventions. *EcoHealth*, 12(4), 560–562. https://doi.org/10.1007/s10393-015-1042-3

Eaton-Stull, Y. M., Jaffe, B., Scott, K., & Shiller, M. (2023). Animal-assisted crisis response: Characteristics of canine handlers and their canine partners. *Human-Animal Interactions*, 11(1), https://doi.org/10.1079/hai.2023.0033

ESPN (2024). A day in the life of Beacon, the therapy dog at the U.S. Olympic gymnastics trials. Retrieved July 10, 2024 from: https://www.espn.com/olympics/gymnastics/story/_/id/40459211/2024-gymnastics-olympic-trials-beacon-therapy-dog-usa

Fournier, A. K. (2019). *Animal-assisted intervention: Thinking empirically.* Cham, Switzerland: Palgrave MacMillian.

Haraway, D. J. (2008). *When species meet.* University of Minnesota Press.

Ng, Z., Albright, J., Fine, A. H., & Peralta, J. (2015). Our ethical and moral responsibility: Ensuring the welfare of therapy animals. In Aubrey H. Fine (Ed.), *Handbook on animal-assisted therapy: Foundations and guidelines for animal-assisted interventions* (4th ed., pp. 91–101). Elsevier/Academic Press.

Pendry, P., & Vandagriff, J. L. (2019). Animal visitation program (AVP) reduces cortisol levels of university students: A randomized controlled trial. *AERA Open*, 5, 1–12. https://doi.org/10.1177/2332858419852592

Peralta, J. M., & Fine, A. H. (2021). *The welfare of animals in animal-assisted interventions: Foundations and best practice methods.* Springer.

Pinillos, R. G. (2018). The path to developing a one welfare framework. *One Welfare: A Framework to Improve Animal Welfare and Human Well-Being*, 1–15. https://doi.org/10.1079/9781786393845.0001

Rodriguez, K. E., Green, F. L. L., Binfet, J. T., Townsend, L., & Gee, N. (2023). Complexities and considerations in conducting animal-assisted intervention research: A discussion of randomized controlled trials. *Human–Animal Interactions*, https://doi.org/10.1079/hai.2023.0004

Shapiro, K. (2020). Human-animal studies: Remembering the past, celebrating the present, troubling the future. *Society & Animals*, 28(7), 797–833. https://doi.org/10.1163/15685306-bja10029

Wagner, C., Grob, C., & Hediger, K. (2022). Specific and non-specific factors of animal-assisted interventions considered in research: A systematic review. *Frontiers in Psychology*, 13, e931347. https://doi.org/10.3389/fpsyg.2022.931347

Williams, J. M., Bradfield, J., Gardiner, A., Pendry, P., & Wauthier, L. (2024). Co-producing Paws on Campus: A psychoeducational dog-facilitated programme for university students experiencing mental health difficulties. *International Journal of Environmental Research and Public Health*, 21, 1066. https://doi.org/10.3390/ijerph21081066

Index

Note: **Bold** page numbers refer to tables, *italic* page numbers refer to figures.

For Product Safety Concerns and Information please contact our EU
representative GPSR@taylorandfrancis.com
Taylor & Francis Verlag GmbH, Kaufingerstraße 24, 80331 München, Germany

www.ingramcontent.com/pod-product-compliance
Lightning Source LLC
Chambersburg PA
CBHW050643280326
41932CB00015B/2758